Systemic Lupus Erythematosus

Systemic Lupus Erythematosus

Marian W. Ropes

Harvard University Press, Cambridge, Massachusetts
and London, England   1976

Copyright © 1976 by the President and Fellows of Harvard College
All rights reserved
Printed in the United States of America

Library of Congress Cataloging in Publication Data

Ropes, Marian Wilkins, 1903-
    Systemic lupus erythematosus.

    Bibliography: p.
    Includes index.
    1. Lupus erythematosus, Systemic. I. Title. [DNLM: 1. Lupus erythemato-
sus, Systemic. WR152   R785s]
RC924.R66   616.7'7   75-31988
ISBN 0-674-86255-4

Preface

Systemic lupus erythematosus is a disease of unknown etiology whose course is still not generally known and concerning which no consensus exists as to the proper treatment. The Arthritis Unit at the Massachusetts General Hospital has been interested in SLE since the formation of the group forty-five years ago. Because of the fortunate combination of available hospital beds, a weekly follow-up clinic and an effective follow-up system, study of patients with SLE has been possible over long periods of time. Many of the patients were first seen in consultation in the hospital and then followed in the Arthritis Clinic. In addition, the individual physicians of the unit have followed many lupus patients in their offices. In this setting my interest in SLE started over forty years ago and has been fostered by an apparently higher incidence and an increasing knowledge of the disease. Very disturbing to me has been the general failure to realize the great variety of courses and thus the inability to estimate the prognosis in any one case. However, my greatest concern has been the diverse treatments, often toxic, supported by many investigators without evidence as to the value of the treatments. Equally unfortunate is the lack of knowledge of the beneficial effect of a conservative regimen.

With this background, I present my experience with the disease, based not only on the 142 patients in whom the findings have been analyzed statistically, but also on the many other patients seen by me. The number has increased in frequency in recent years. There has been no statistical study of patients seen since 1966.

The present study is based on patients seen either on the wards or in the outpatient clinics of the Massachusetts General Hospital or in offices of the members of the Arthritis Unit between the years 1932 and 1966. Many were first admitted to the Dermatological and Neurological services, and all with significant renal disease were seen by the Renal Group. Data on the original group of patients were collected in 1938 and enlarged and reviewed in 1949. They have been analyzed separately in some respects and offer an interesting contrast to the series collected in the subsequent 17 years. In general, the second series represents a group of patients seen after steroids were available (though used in only 72% of the cases), and after antibiotics of wide effectiveness were used. Perhaps of even greater significance is the fact that in this group the likelihood of earlier diagnosis was present because of greater awareness of the early, mild stages of the disease, use of the determination of the presence of "LE" cells and antinuclear antibodies to increase suspicion of the disease, and realization of the possible implication of lupus by the presence of false positive serology for syphilis.

The series analyzed has one or more of the following advantages over the majority of other published series. The diagnostic criteria are strict and clearly defined; positive LE cell tests were not required for diagnosis; the number of patients is larger than that in many series; the follow-up period is longer; and consequently the manifestations and course of the disease are more adequately indicated.

The presentation of this material cannot solve the many questions that persist concerning systemic lupus erythematosus. However, it gives a more complete picture of the course of the disease, and offers indications of the value of a general conservative regimen. It indicates the reason I prefer to use this regimen with aspirin as the anti-inflammatory agent whenever possible, rather than to depend on the more toxic anti-inflammatory drugs.

I am indebted to the members of the Medical Service of the Massachusetts General Hospital who allowed the inclusion of their patients in this series. I wish to thank Drs. Kurt Bloch, Stephen Krane, Lawrence Miller, John Mills, and Charles Short, members of the Arthritis Unit, for reading portions of the text. The collection and analysis of the material were carried out with the assistance of Miss Hope Richardson and Mrs. Cynthia Krane. I am indebted to Mrs. Anne Sullivan for secretarial assistance, and to Mrs. Eleanor Pyle for help in editing the manuscript. Grants from the Massachusetts Chapter of the Arthritis Foundation aided in the preparation of the book.

Boston, Massachusetts   Marian W. Ropes

Contents

Systemic Lupus Erythematosus

1 History and Classification

The first recognition of systemic lupus erythematosus (SLE) as a disease entity is usually ascribed to Kaposi in 1872 [126]. He noted two types: one with acute or subacute eruption often preceded by joint pain and swelling and associated with lymph node enlargement; the second with severe diffuse redness and swelling, a typhoid-like state, pleurisy and pneumonia, sometimes mental disturbances, and often death in 2 to 3 weeks but remission in some cases. Osler [195] in 1904 described patients who undoubtedly had SLE in his erythema group of skin diseases, and placed further emphasis on the systemic nature of the disease. Keil [127] in 1937 concluded that acute and discoid lupus erythematosus were related.

Notable pathological changes were described by Libman and Sacks [153] in 1924. Outstanding was the recognition and description of the verrucous lesions on the valves of the heart. Hematoxylin bodies were first described by Gross [92] in 1932. Baehr et al. [15], in an extensive clinical and pathological study of the disease, first described wire-loop lesions in the glomeruli in 1935.

Characteristic laboratory findings were reported later. The "LE cell" was first described by Hargraves et al. in 1948 [101]. The presence of LE cells in patients treated with hydralazine was described in 1954. Their occurrence with other therapy and in other diseases was subsequently noted by many [73, 156, 197, 237, 285]. Moore and Lutz [185] proved the frequency of false positive tests for syphilis in patients with SLE, and noted the presence of this result years before the appearance of the clinical picture of SLE. Lessened activity of complement in the blood of patients with SLE was found by Elliott and Mathieson in 1953 [76]. Antibodies to DNA were demonstrated in 1957 (see review by Arana and Seligman, [10], and in 1966 Tan et al. [262] reported the presence of DNA itself in the blood. Deposition of γ globulin and complement has been noted in glomeruli [123, 150, 175], skin [41, 202, 261, 272], choroid plexus [14], and synovial tissues since 1957 [36], and DNA in glomeruli since 1967 [134].

Systemic lupus erythematosus is one of a large group of relatively common clinical entities that involve many systems—the "generalized connective tissue diseases" or "collagen diseases." Not only is the etiology of these entities unknown and the pathogenetic mechanisms poorly understood, but the interrelationships between the individual entities remain in question. Clinically there are many similarities despite the clear-cut differences between the fully developed, typical pictures. The associated laboratory abnormalities also present much overlapping even in the factors that suggest some specificity. Pathologically, also, the similarities are notable, in association with a few relatively specific or differentiating tissue changes.

There are differences of opinion as to which clinical entities should be included in this group, but there is general agreement as to the inclusion of rheumatoid arthritis, rheumatic fever, systemic lupus erythematosus, dermatomyositis, scleroderma and, by many investigators, periarteritis nodosa. Many entities or syndromes must be considered as possible members of this group. Outstanding among these are glomerulonephritis; many of the vasculitides in addition to periarteritis nodosa, including hypersensitivity arteritis, Henoch-Schönlein's purpura, Wegener's granuloma, and temporal or giant-cell granulomatous arteritis; erythema multiforme exudativum; Stevens-Johnson syndrome; Behçet's syndrome, and perhaps Whipple's disease.

A suitable name for this group of heterogeneous clinical entities has not been found. The obvious involvement of the intercellular components of connective tissue in many organs focused attention on this tissue system as the apparent site of the diseases. The concept of connective tissue disease was introduced by Klinge [133] in relation to rheumatic fever and rheumatoid arthritis. Klemperer and his colleagues [131] explained the systemic nature of systemic lupus erythematosus in like manner. They, however, stressed the striking alterations in the collagenous component of fibrous connective tissue and coined the term "collagen disease" [132]. They were fully aware that the collagen changes were but one of the morphological characteristics of the underlying morbid disease process. Klemperer made this clear when he wrote the following: "The term, collagen disease, was originally proposed to call attention to systemic alterations of the extracellular components of the connective tissue as a pathologic-anatomic feature common to a group of apparently heterogeneous diseases. It was not intended to use the term in a diagnostic sense, since it was realized that it referred to one morphologic characteristic only, and, therefore, obviously could not define the underlying morbid process of the diseases grouped together." Because the term "collagen disease" implies that the changes occur primarily in collagen fibers, it is misleading. We prefer the more inclusive term, the connective tissue diseases, when referring to this group of disorders, since all components of connective tissue are involved. This term, though convenient, is arbitrary and not really satisfactory. Like others in use, it gives no indication of the extensive, often marked, vascular involvement present in these disorders. Perhaps we must await further knowledge of the etiology or pathogenesis and of interrelationships between the various entities before a suitable name can be found.

In fully developed form, each individual disease presents a picture so characteristic that diagnosis can be made readily with relative certainty. Early, mild, or atypical cases may present a great problem in diagnosis, however, and since there is no proof of the diagnosis in any of these diseases, real difference of opinion may exist concerning individual patients. As a result there may be little uniformity in the cases included under any of the diagnostic labels. Therefore, in the study and analysis of any of the diseases, it is essential to have criteria whereby the limits of each disease entity are determined, and whereby it may be apparent to all just what cases are included in each diagnostic classification. Only in this way can the knowledge of one group in regard to these diseases be compared with and added to that of other groups. And also only in this way can we hope to recognize clues from the natural history of these diseases that may lead to more profitable explanations as to the etiology or pathogenetic mechanisms or interrelationships or proof of diagnosis.

Systemic lupus erythematosus is readily recognized when the characteristic manifestations are present. The concurrence of a typical rash in butterfly distribution with atrophy and follicular plugging, mild arthritis, serositis, albuminuria and hematuria, leukopenia and severe anemia would leave little doubt that the patient had disseminated lupus. However, if the diagnosis is limited to such situations, only the severe and usually the late cases will be recognized. It is now generally accepted that patients may have mild disease with only a few of these characteristic manifestations for many years. During this period definite diagnosis is often impossible except in retrospect, though it may be suspected if LE cells or false-positive serological tests for syphilis are found, and to a lesser extent if antinuclear antibodies are present in the blood.

Though there is general knowledge of the features that characterize patients with typical systemic lupus erythematosus, no tested and accepted specific criteria for classification existed until recently [51]. The literature is replete with articles containing excellent information in regard to the disease and its manifestations, often well illustrated or tabulated, but few have delineated the limits of the diagnosis accurately enough to enable other investigators to know just what cases are included in the groups discussed, or to relate the course to various manifestations or one manifestation to another. Fortunately, criteria for classification of the disease and delineation of the limits acceptable for the diagnosis of definite SLE have been compiled and tested by a committee of the American Rheumatism Association [51]. It will now be possible to compare the series of various investigators to obtain more accurate knowledge of manifestations, course, and effect of treatment. The criteria have already been tested by several groups, with good agreement [154, 269].

Classification and Criteria

In the present series the clinical findings used in selecting patients were four:
1. Skin rash: persistent erythema over cheeks and nose; or erythematous lesions with atrophy and follicular plugging anywhere.
2. Kidney involvement with albuminuria and/or hematuria in the absence of infection or amyloidosis.
3. Serositis.
4. Joint involvement.

For inclusion in the study, a patient must have manifested 3 of the 4 above criteria or have both 1 and 2. The presence, in addition, of a leukopenia; severe anemia (below 8 gm per 100 ml), especially with evidence of hemolysis; thrombocytopenia; false-positive serological test for syphilis; significant hair loss; palpable spleen; palpable liver; telangiectasia along edges of eyelids or at bases of nails; patchy pneumonitis with atelectasis; psychosis; or seizures would certainly help support the diagnosis, but none of these alone led to the classification of patients as having disseminated lupus. Similarly, no patients were classified as systemic lupus if they had LE cells in the blood but did not satisfy the above criteria. All of the patients included in the series would satisfy the criteria adopted by the American Rheumatism Association for classification of patients with SLE [51].

For this study the patients were classified first by the above criteria into three groups: I, classical: patients with both 1 and 2 of the criteria; II, definite: patients with either 1 or 2 of the criteria and 3 and 4; and III, possible: patients with only 2 of the criteria, not including both 1 and 2. Patients falling into the first two groups (classical and definite) would be considered by almost all clinicians to have systemic lupus erythematosus. In the third group the usual difficulty in differential diagnosis was in deciding between lupus and another of the generalized connective tissue diseases. In some cases, the likelihood of lupus was great but the evidence not quite strong enough to include the patients in the definite group. Many of these who presented a picture strongly suggestive of lupus also would be diagnosed by the majority of physicians as systemic lupus. In addition, the groups classified by the above criteria were compared with groups delineated by the final clinical diagnosis made at the time the patient was studied. These diagnoses represent the consensus of opinion of the physicians caring for the patients, including those in the Arthritis Unit, and agree closely with the classification by the criteria in the study. In classification no consideration was given to the presence or absence of LE cells or rheumatoid factor, each group being subsequently divided by these factors, if available, and compared. Analyses of groups I and II will be presented in this book.

Degrees of Activity

For the purposes of comparison and classification, the activity of SLE in each patient was classified into grades 1, 2, 3, and 4, and the course of each patient charted in these terms. Grade 1 represents rather minimal activity, as manifested by various combinations of symptoms and signs (Tables 1 and 2). Grade 2 indicates greater activity of the disease, with a greater degree of any of the symptoms and signs and occasionally slight fever. Fatiguability or other symptoms often limit activities. Grade 3 represents marked activity of the disease. Any of the symptoms or signs may be marked. Grade 4 indicates a potentially moribund state, often with lethargy, and severe involvement of any system. The case reports (see Appendix) and accompanying figures indicate the way in which the grades of activity were estimated.

"Crisis" in SLE is used to designate extremely severe activity of the disease. It is similar to grade 3 to 4 activity. Before adequate antibiotic and corticosteroid therapy were available, lupus crisis resulted in death in a high percentage of cases. It was the cause of death in 40% compared to death from infection in 40% and from renal failure in 14% of the 62 cases seen before 1949. Lupus crisis when fully developed is usually manifested by high fever (which may rise to 106° F or more), extreme generalized weakness and fatigue, severe headache, marked abdominal pain, and often chest pain. It may be accompanied by severe involvement of various systems with, for instance, myocarditis and cardiac failure, or cerebral manifestations often with seizures, psychosis or coma. It is frequently complicated by severe infections, either localized or with septicemia. Renal involvement, if present, is often intensified, with resulting severe failure, but rarely is of significance in early disease presenting in crisis.

Laboratory findings confirm the severity of SLE in crisis. Hemoglobin not uncommonly falls to 5 gm or less per 100 ml, leukocyte count usually is below 2,000 per cu mm, platelet count falls occasionally to 2,500 per cu mm, sedimentation rate is markedly elevated, and complement levels, especially C'3, are usually low. In the experience of Schur and Sandson [226], high titers of complement-fixing antibod-

Table 1. Clinical manifestations of grades 1, 2, 3, and 4 activity. Any systems may be involved in any combination.

Degree of activity	Malaise and fatiguability	Morning stiffness	Rash	Hair loss	Joint involvement
Grade 1	0 to slight	0 to slight	occasional slight	±	arthralgia
Grade 2	slight to moderate	slight to moderate	slight to moderate	±	some arthritis
Grade 3	moderate to marked	moderate to marked	moderate to marked	moderate	moderate arthritis
Grade 4	marked	marked	marked	often severe	marked arthritis

ies to DNA are usually present. Urinary findings vary. In the acute, early cases albuminuria may be slight (1 to 2+), red cells in the urine only slightly above normal, and white cells low or in some cases markedly elevated even in the absence of infection. In later cases, renal failure may supervene rapidly with blood urea nitrogen (BUN) rising above 100 mg/100 ml and associated urinary changes of marked albuminuria (4+) and increased red cells and white cells with cellular casts.

Despite increasing knowledge of mechanisms involved in SLE, still little is known of its fundamental nature, not enough of the extreme variations in manifestations and course, and distressingly little of the effect of treatment or of the treatment to be recommended. The disease is seen more commonly than thirty years ago and the mortality is much lower than previously realized. However, it remains a serious illness with a surprising tendency to sudden, acute, occasionally fatal exacerbations precipitated by a wide variety of factors. The better prognosis makes it essential to recognize the disease as soon as possible and to determine the regimen which lessens the tendency to acute exacerbations and under which remission occurs.

Obviously the answers to many of the questions await the results of investigations of the present and even the future, but better acquaintance with the nature, characteristics, influencing factors, course, treatment, and final state will in itself make more secure the diagnosis, improve the handling of patients, and alter the pessimistic attitude toward the disease.

Fever, °F (rectal)	Pleural or pericardial pain	Mouth ulcers	Headache	Abdominal pain	Convulsions, psychosis, or coma
0	0	0	0	0	0
occasional slight	occasional slight	slight	0	0	0
up to 102	moderate	moderate	±	±	±
up to 107	often marked	often marked	often severe	often severe	often severe

Table 2. Laboratory findings in grades 1, 2, 3, and 4 activity; any systems may be involved in any combination.

Degree of activity	Hematocrit (%)	Leucocyte count (per cu mm)	Platelet count (per cu mm)	Sedimentation rate [1] (mm/min)
Grade 1	36 ±	4,000 ±	normal	up to 0.5
Grade 2	32 ±	3,000 ±	occasionally reduced	0.8
Grade 3	28 ±	2,000 ±	< 100,000	1.5
Grade 4	20	< 2,000	< 40,000	2.0

[1] By the method of Rourke and Ernstene [217] the upper limit or normal is 0.35 mm/min.

Incidence

Systemic lupus erythematosus is seen more commonly than it was thirty or forty years ago, but it is difficult to determine whether it really occurs more frequently or is merely better recognized. Surely many cases are diagnosed earlier because of realization of the many modes of onset and recognition of the fact that the course may be mild and of long duration. However, review of the cases in this series that were first seen before 1949 reveals that 82% were acute in onset and, therefore, probably did not remain undiagnosed through a long period of mild disease. Earlier recognition of cases has been increased also by realization of the possible significance of a false-positive serological reaction for syphilis, and by the stimulus produced by a positive LE cell test to attempt to corroborate the diagnosis, even in early cases. But to those of us who have been attempting to make this diagnosis for the past thirty-five or forty years there seem now to be even more of the typical cases, in addition to the early, mild, or atypical ones discovered in the manners just discussed.

The actual incidence remains unknown. Various estimates have been made but are hard to evaluate. Svanborg [258] in 1957 had noticed an increase, from 3 cases treated in 1938 and 1939 and 3 in 1948 and 1949, to 18 in 1954 and 1955 in a population of 380,000. These fig-

Albumin in urine	Red cells in urine	White cells in urine	BUN (mg/100 ml)	Creatinine clearance (liter/24 hr)
	per high-power field			
often 1 +	usually normal	usually normal	normal	normal
2 +	> 10	> 20	occasional slight elevation	occasional slight reduction
3 to 4 +	often > 20 with red-cell casts	often > 30 with white-cell casts	50 ±	90 or less
4 +	often > 20 with red-cell casts	often > 30 with white-cell casts	100 +	40 or less

ures would correlate with Leonhardt's statement in 1964 [149] of 1 overt case in 8,000 persons, and perhaps with Siegel's figure in 1965 [238] of 2.6 in 100,000 annually and Cross's figure in 1960 [60] of 15 to 20 cases a year in 40,000 outpatient visits.

Etiology

The etiology of systemic lupus erythematosus remains unknown, even though many of the pathogenetic mechanisms are partially understood. Its essential nature has not been elucidated, nor has the extent, if any, to which hereditary factors play a role. Two major hypotheses are generally considered: 1) that immune alterations represent the fundamental etiology of SLE; and 2) that the underlying cause is infection with a virus or other as yet unrecognized organism.

Rapidly increasing knowledge continues to provide more and more evidence of the abnormalities of immune phenomena in the disease. Well-documented are the decreased levels of complement components [76, 115, 225]; the almost universal presence of antinuclear antibodies [10, 20, 166, 216, 256], including those to nucleoprotein, DNA, and histone; the presence of the antinuclear factor that leads to formation of LE cells by the sera of 85 to 90% of SLE patients; the finding of antibodies to native and denatured DNA, and, at periods in the disease, free DNA in the blood [10, 44, 113, 226, 262]; the relatively specific finding of antibodies to double-stranded DNA [201] and to double-stranded RNA [227]; and increased serum concentrations of immuno-globulins [20, 45, 87, 225]. Further evidence of the immune alterations includes the occurrence of thrombocytopenia and hemolytic anemia, often with positive Coombs' test; and the presence of cold-precipitable complexes (cryoproteins) [160, 249]. Many of the alterations found in SLE are in no way specific and it is intriguing that some, like hemo-lytic anemia, thyroiditis, and Sjögren's syndrome, are found in rheu-matioid arthritis. Even LE cells have been reported in 4 to 27% of pa-tients with rheumatoid arthritis [11, 81, 100, 108, 148, 268]. In our experience they are found in 6%. Deposition of DNA in glomeruli [134] and of γ globulin and complement components in glomeruli [123, 150, 175], in the skin [41, 58, 202, 261, 272], in the choroid plexus [14], and in the synovial tissues [36] has been demonstrated in SLE.

Nevertheless, proof that any of the factors that are increased in the blood or deposited in tissues lead to the overall disease, SLE, is lack-ing. There is little question that they are implicated in the pathogenetic mechanisms that produce signs and symptoms of the disease, and that much of the inflammatory process is associated with the deposition of complexes of antigen, antibody, and complement. However, there is no proof that they represent the fundamental etiology [275].

A correlation of the levels of various proteins in the serum with activity of the disease has been observed, especially with complement components and anti-DNA antibodies [20, 87, 112, 226]. Abnormali-ties in any of these have been considered as indication for treatment with such agents as corticosteroids or immunosuppressive drugs, regardless of the clinical state of the patient. However, the many exceptions to a complete correlation of the serum factors with the clin-ical activity make any such rule for treatment very unwise. There is not adequate evidence that the serological findings indicate prognosis. Occasionally in our experience severe, active SLE may progress stead-ily to death in the presence of normal whole hemolytic complement and normal or slightly low C3 levels.

Suggestion of hereditary factors is slight. Incidence of 2 or 3 cases in a family is being reported more frequently and was seen in 3 of our cases but the total familial incidence is still not high, approximately 150 cases [12, 40, 69, 94]. The patients reported in the literature include 14 pairs of concordant identical twins and 2 pairs of heterologous twins. It is probable that one should not include the cases of "neonatal lupus" which, in general, have had skin rash confirmed by biopsy in some cases or LE cells or both. The mothers of all but one of the reported cases have had definite SLE, either before or after the birth of the child [28, 37, 69, 77, 116, 171, 177, 192, 229]. The signs in the babies have been assumed to be due to placental passage of the LE factor (a 7S globulin). In most babies the rash and LE cells have disappeared within a few months. In at least 2 cases the signs persisted for several months. One child in whom the diagnosis was questionable died at the age of 4 [192].

In the present series one baby born prematurely at 8 months while the mother had active lupus lived only 13 hours. Laboratory examinations showed hematocrit of 30%, leukocyte count of 5,650, positive Coombs test, and LE cells in the blood. The findings were strongly suggestive of SLE. However, at postmortem examination there were no definite changes of lupus. There were extensive hemorrhages in the lungs, intraventricular hemorrhage, and many petechiae on the skin. The spleen showed some periarteriolar laminar thickening. Another child born to the same mother when her disease was less active has very small kidneys and severe renal failure at the age of 3. Her physicians doubt that this abnormality is due to lupus. In a stillborn baby of another patient who had active lupus, postmortem examination showed petechial hemorrhages in the epicardium and pleurae. One other child in this series whose mother had active lupus was reported by the mother to have developed a rash over cheeks and nose after being exposed to the sun at the age of 4 months.

The increased incidence of elevated γ globulins in families of patients with SLE is difficult to interpret. Studies are few, inconsistent, and limited in range [9, 83, 149, 207, 238, 266]. The possibility that the elevation of globulin is associated with subclinical disease or a period of remission must be considered.

The second hypothesis as to the fundamental etiology of SLE, the one I favor, is that the underlying cause is infection with a virus or other as yet unrecognized organism. Inherent in this theory is the belief that the alterations in immunological reactions known to occur in SLE can be produced by an infectious agent. One such occurrence, not understood, is the production in syphilis of an "antibody" producing the Wassermann or similar reaction with tissue antigen. There is no known direct relationship to the spirochete. Of great interest is the fact that the same reaction is found as a "false-positive" test in 10 to

20% of patients with SLE [57, 60, 109, 137, 159]. The immunological basis of poststreptococcal glomerulonephritis is more apparent, and may correspond to part of the tissue changes in SLE presumably caused by immune complexes. Other evidence of altered immune reactions to infection has been reported [23, 286]. The possible role of the combination of a virus infection and abnormal immune reactions in the etiology of SLE was discussed by Ziff [284], Talal and Steinberg [260], and Schur et al. [227].

However, for the theory that an infection causes SLE there is as yet no evidence. Virus-like bodies have been noted in tissues since the report by Györkey et al. [96]; see review by Grimley et al. [91]. There is no substantiation yet of their pathogenetic significance. The increased incidence of antibodies to viruses, especially the paramyxoma virus, is difficult to interpret [124, 284], but can lead to speculation that a virus infection plays a role [227, 284]. The similarity of SLE to virus-induced animal diseases is circumstantial evidence [72, 174, 284].

The sex incidence in SLE, with marked predominance of females, gives no real support for one hypothesis over the other. The tendency for complete remissions with disappearance of all signs and symptoms, and then with recurrence in some cases, would perhaps be better explained on the basis of an infectious process. The LE cell factor may or may not persist in such remissions. Improvement in the disease with rest is also more consistent with an infectious etiology and corresponds with the situation in many known infections.

2 Characteristics, Manifestations, and Pathologic Findings

The description of the characteristics found in the present series will represent those found in the classical and definite groups (Groups I and II) combined. When indicated they will be compared with those of other generalized connective-tissue diseases. It seems of little value to compare extensively the individual findings with those in the many series reported. The majority of the series suffer from at least one of three common defects: 1) a lack of description of clear-cut criteria on which the diagnosis is based; 2) the common errors of either including only patients in whom the LE cell tests are positive or, equally unwisely, including all patients who have positive LE cell tests despite the lack of characteristic clinical pictures; 3) too small a series of patients with too short a follow-up. Therefore no detailed table will be added to those in the literature (such as those in *11, 24, 55, 60, 69, 78, 102, 103, 106, 119, 183, 216, 220*). However, our results will be presented and in discussing the incidence of the findings in this series, indication will be given as to the extent to which they agree with those in other series. A preliminary report on part of this series was published in 1964 [*208*]. Postmortem examinations were performed in 58 patients, 49 females and 9 males. The neuropathological findings on 19 of these patients were described by Johnson and Richardson [*121*].

The Patient Series

Sex

The present series of 142 consists of 18 males (13%) and 124 females (87%). A similar markedly increased prevalence of systemic lupus in females has been reported by all other investigators, though the percentage varies slightly. The mode of selection of the patients for this study should not have favored inclusion of either sex.

Race

Information on racial background was available for 134 of the patients in our series. Of these 46% (60) were from countries in the Mediterranean latitudes, including Italy (41 patients), Greece (8), and Portugal (7); 1 patient was from the West Indies. All other countries provided only 54% (73).

Table 3. The racial background of the 134 patients for whom information was available.

Nationality or race	Number of patients
Mediterranean countries	
Italy	41
Greece	8
Portugal	7
Other	4
West Indies	1
Caucasian from countries other than Mediterranean	70
Black	2
Oriental	1

This distribution is in great contrast to that found in the group of patients with rheumatoid arthritis studied at the time the first quarter of this series was seen [234]. In the rheumatoid group 7% (21) were of Italian origin, and 93% (272) from countries above the latitudes described. The distribution in the present series may correspond to that found by Siegel [239], which suggested an increased prevalence of blacks and Puerto Ricans in New York City in those dying of SLE but not in those dying of periarteritis, and to the higher incidence of SLE found in black than in white males discharged from veterans' hospitals [238].

Familial Incidence

Occurrence of more than one case in a family has been reported by many investigators (see review by Brunjes [40]) but the total number of families involved is not high, approximately 75, with 14 sets of concordant identical twins [12, 69, 82, 88, 94, 103, 122, 244, 266]. In our series of 142 cases, three families had more than one case of SLE. In the family of one other patient there was a questionable case. In one of these families, two sisters have had the disease. One is in good remission after 9 years but the other had severe renal disease and died 10 years after onset. In another family, father and daughter had SLE; the daughter was ill first and died in 3⅓ years; the father is in almost complete remission after 12 years. In the third family, two sisters and two brothers were involved; the two brothers and one sister have died after 8 to 10 years of disease and the other sister is in good remission after 23 years, including 7 years since the series was closed. In the fourth family, one woman had typical disease and died after 19 years. A sister was told that a facial rash was "lupus" but she was not seen by us. One other family in which two sisters had SLE has been seen since the series was closed. The findings in newborn babies of mothers with SLE have been discussed.

Family History

A family history of joint disease was reported in 31% of the 124 cases in which information was available. However, the type of disease was unknown in most instances, so the significance of this high percentage is not determinable. In the series of patients with rheumatoid arthritis reported by Short and Bauer [234], the family history of joint disease was 47%, 12% representing rheumatic fever. In the present series the family history represented rheumatic fever in 8%.

The Disease

Type of Disease

Entirely typical disease with involvement of both skin and kidneys occurred in 68% (97 of 142) of the present series. In the remaining cases, the clinical picture was characteristic with involvement of skin or kidneys, and other manifestations as discussed under criteria.

Age of Onset

The ages of onset of the disease in this series occurred over a wide range which was similar to that recorded by other investigators. In the majority of cases, 61% (87 of 142), onset occurred between the ages of 15 and 30, and in 47% (67 of 142) between 15 and 24. Six percent (9) had onset at 50 or later, and only 8% (11) before 15, a somewhat lower incidence in children than in other series (the source of patients under 15 was limited in this series). The range in ages, 4 to 72 years, was, however, comparable to that in other groups.

Some differences in age of onset in different series would be expected because of the difference of opinion in deciding what to accept as the onset. The decision in the majority of cases is simple, since the first symptoms or signs are followed, more or less steadily, by enough other manifestations to make the diagnosis definite. However, exceptions are common and often the decision as to the time of onset cannot be made with assurance—for instance, when an episode of hemolytic anemia or thrombocytopenia (without obvious causative factor) occurs many months or years before the appearance, after a symptom-free period, of more definitive symptoms or signs. In the few cases of this type in the present series, the attack of hemolytic anemia has usually been considered to be the onset of the disease. However, in instances in which the first illness was not as specific, or the likely possibility of other causative factors could not be ruled out, it was not considered to be the onset. In the majority of these latter cases, the first illness was joint disease, entirely consistent with the joint involvement of disseminated lupus but surely indistinguishable by history from that of other diseases, such as rheumatoid arthritis or often even rheumatic fever. The high incidence in our series of such previous joint disease—16% (21) in the 133 cases in whom information was available—occurring 10 to 50 years before the onset of typical systemic lupus is of great interest. It seems probable that in many cases the joint involvement represented the onset of lupus. If so, the group of patients in whom disease started before 15 years of age would increase from 8% (11) to 14% (20). In addition, the average duration of disease would be increased markedly (as discussed later). There was no correlation between the age of onset and the systems first involved.

Type of Onset

In 30% (43) of the series of 142 the onset was acute. An arbitrary definition of acute onset was the progression to grade 2 severity within 2 months. This type of onset is shown in cases 3, 6, 11, and 12 (Appendix). Often the progression occurred in a few hours. The frequency of such onset was not affected by age, racial background, the degree to which the disease was typical, sex, past history of joint disease, infections, sensitivity to sun or drugs, rash, number of joints subsequently involved, loss of hair, psychosis, convulsions, fever, nodules, hepatomegaly, splenomegaly, hemoglobin concentration, white cell count, degree of albuminuria, hematuria, casts, urea nitrogen concentration, prolongation of P-R intervals, T-wave abnormalities, or positive serological tests for syphilis.

However, the type of onset showed marked correlation with the system first involved ($p = 0.002$). Eighty-nine percent (25) of the 28 patients with skin involvement as the first sign had gradual onset, in contrast to 39% (12) of the 31 in whom several systems were initially involved. Of the patients with acute onset, 7% (3 of 43) had skin involvement first, and 46% (20 of 43) had several systems involved at the onset, in contrast to 27% (27 of 99) and 13% (13 of 99) respectively in the patients in whom the onset was gradual. The percentage of patients with joint or systemic involvement first was similar in the groups of acute and gradual onset.

Acute onset was not seen in any of the 12 patients who had negative tests for LE cells, whereas 39% (29) of the 75 with positive tests had acute onset ($p = 0.02$).

Very slight correlation was present between the Coombs test and the type of onset ($p = 0.19$). Forty-four percent (8) of the 18 patients with positive tests had acute onset in contrast to 26% (11) of the 42 with negative tests.

System First Involved

Consistent with the great variation in the disease from patient to patient is the difference in type of onset, in so far as the system first involved is concerned. Joint involvement was the first manifestation in 27% (38 of 142) of the patients of this series; systemic symptoms, including fever, weight loss, fatiguability and weakness, in 25% (36 of 142); involvement of several systems at once in 22% (31 of 142); skin rash in 20% (28 of 142), with 13% (18) having facial rash only at the onset; and other systems (such as pleura or hematopoietic system) in 6% (9 of 142). The distribution of systems first involved is similar to that reported by other workers [69, 102, 103]. The high incidence of joint involvement at the onset could be related to the fact that this series was followed by physicians active in the treatment of rheumatic diseases, though many of the cases were first seen by members of the Dermatology or General Medical services and referred to the Arthritis

Unit. However, even higher incidences were found by others [69, 102, 103, 106].

When only one system is first involved (whether it be joints or skin or other) it may remain the only manifestation of disease for months or years. In this series the longest period during which only joints, with or without systemic symptoms, were involved before the characteristic total picture developed was 14 years, with an interval of 1 year or more in 12 of the 97 patients in whom information was available. Similarly long intervals, up to 31 years, were found in 21 patients with skin involvement as the first symptom. This includes discoid lesions as one stage of systemic lupus in 16 of 97 patients. Such intervals in the patients with discoid lesions were as long as 22 years, during which time the only possible diagnosis was discoid lupus, but these were followed by typical systemic lupus erythematosus.

Factors Causing Exacerbation

Outstanding in the histories of patients with SLE, and extremely troublesome in the treatment of these patients, is the ease with which exacerbations of disease may be precipitated by various factors [69, 186]. Most common among these are infections, emotional or physical stress, sun sensitivity, operations, pregnancy, and drugs.

Infection

Infections occurred in 79% (108) of the 137 patients on whom information was available. In 86 of these, the presence or absence of exacerbation following the infection could be determined and 85% (73) suffered exacerbations. In many patients in this series, exacerbations of SLE occurred on several occasions after various infections, but in approximately the same number of patients exacerbations occurred only after one infection and not after others. In some cases it is difficult to determine whether infection is present or whether the signs and symptoms suggesting infection represent an exacerbation of SLE, or whether both infection and exacerbation of SLE are present. Proof can be obtained only by cultures or in occasional patients by response to antibiotic therapy.

There is some evidence in our series that the patients with lupus had more frequent infections [191], as has been suggested by others [248], and there is very strong indication that they had exacerbations with infections, and also a clinical impression that they handled infections less well than other patients. The difficulty may in fact represent an inadequate reaction to the infection because of the flare of the underlying disease with its known effect on the immune mechanism [23, 260].

Blood cultures were positive in 19 of the 69 patients from whom they were obtained. In the majority of cases the septicemia occurred terminally but it was not uncommon in severe exacerbations. In 2 patients there was subacute bacterial endocarditis. In 2 cases the septicemia was associated with severe cellulitis. Extensive decubitus ulcers occurred in 5 cases. The most commonly occurring organism in blood cultures was Staphylococcus aureus (in 7 patients), but a and β hemolytic streptococci, coliform bacilli, pneumococci, H. influenzae, and micrococci were found, and in 1 patient, Cryptococcus neoformans. Meningitis occurred terminally in 2 cases, caused by cryptococcus in 1 case, and a hemolytic streptococcus in the other. Two of the patients have died of meningitis since the series was closed, the organisms being meningococcus and pneumococcus. Osteomyelitis of a vertebra due to salmonella was present in 1 patient and was satisfactorily treated. Perforation of a corneal ulcer, thought due to herpes simplex, occurred in 1 patient receiving 30 mg of prednisone daily. In addition to the septicemias, the infections associated with and presumably producing the exacerbations of lupus were 126 respiratory, including 39 with pneumonia and 12 with otitis media, 18 skin abscesses, 17 herpes zoster, and 41 genitourinary. Single cases of infectious arthritis, infected tenosynovitis, puerperal sepsis, retroperitoneal abscess, measles, and hepatitis occurred. In general the organisms were the common pathogens, especially staphylococci, streptococci, and viruses. Occasionally, however, fortuitous infections with less common organisms occurred, as in the patient with salmonella osteomyelitis, one with moniliasis, and one, seen since the series ended, with cryptococcus infection.

Emotional or Physical Stress

Emotional or physical stress was recognized in 71% (62) of the 87 patients on whom information was available. Of the 45 in whom the presence or absence of exacerbation could be determined, 91% (41) had exacerbations following the stress. The indication of tremendous reactivity to emotional stress with flare of disease, occurring in almost all patients having such stress, corroborates our clinical impression

and that of some other physicians [103, 183, 186]. The "fragility" of
the lupus patients is again apparent. Avoidance of such stress to any
extent possible, and help for the patient in handling his reactivity,
become two major elements in therapy, as will be discussed later.

Operations

   Operations caused exacerbations in many of the patients in this
series, though a complete analysis of the incidence was not made. In
126 operations about which information was available, exacerbations
occurred in 29 patients (23%), usually within a few days but occasionally after a few weeks. In some cases, the procedures were major,
such as hysterectomy, and subtotal gastrectomy. Sympathectomy
(dorsal or lumbar) was followed by exacerbation in 2 patients in the
series. One patient died 6 months after sympathectomy on one side
and 5 months after that on the other side. Her course up to the time of
the first sympathectomy was mild, with a duration of 2½ years and a
severity of grade 2 or less at all times. In 1 other patient initial onset of
the disease apparently started 5 to 8 months after sympathectomy.
However, flare of the disease occurred after even tooth extractions in
3 cases, and after skin and muscle or lymph node biopsies in 5 others.
Similarly, Dubois [69] reported exacerbation after tendon transplant.
Renal biopsy was followed by exacerbation in the 2 patients in this
series on whom biopsies were performed. In one of these death occurred 17 days after a second renal biopsy was made necessary because
inadequate tissue was obtained at the first biopsy. Severe exacerbation
of SLE occurred 4 days after the second biopsy with fever of 104° and
severe lethargy. The serum nonprotein nitrogen (NPN) at that time
was only 45 mg per 100 ml. One week later generalized convulsions
occurred, followed by shock, coma, and subsequently decerebrate
rigidity and death. The relative insignificance of the renal disease as
compared to that of the central nervous system was made more apparent by the fact that the kidneys at postmortem examination
showed only focal lesions in scattered glomeruli. Postmortem examination of the brain showed many small hemorrhages, hyalinization
and fibrinoid necrosis, and infiltration of the adventitia in small and
medium sized arteries, and widespread patchy loss of neurones. In the
other patient in whom exacerbation followed renal biopsy, rash,
fever, and a decrease in renal function occurred in 10 days and the
course was steadily downhill to death 8 weeks after the biopsy.
Splenectomy was associated with an exacerbation in only 2 patients,

in contrast to the findings by Dameshek [63], Dubois [69] and Johnson [120]. It is obviously impossible to determine with certainty that the increased activity of lupus that was noted after any operation was due to the procedure, but the relatively frequent occurrence makes it likely that there is a causal relationship. Avoidance of operative procedures, even minor ones, is wise whenever possible, as will be discussed under therapy.

Pregnancy

Pregnancy is generally accepted as one of the factors that may cause exacerbation of SLE. In the 71 of the women in this series on whom adequate information was available, there was a total of 82 pregnancies, 13 of which ended by spontaneous abortion and 2 by therapeutic interruption. A similar abnormally high frequency of spontaneous abortions has been noted by others [64, 77, 152, 176]. Exacerbation occurred with 38% (27) of the 82 pregnancies, including flares after 5 miscarriages and 1 Caesarian section. Other investigators have noted similar though slightly lower incidence, as summarized by Dubois [64].

The exacerbations varied greatly. In some cases, there was only slight to moderate fever, fatiguability, increased rash including oral lesions, or arthritis, or chest pain or decreased hemoglobin or leukopenia, or a slight increase in albuminuria. In others, the flare consisted of greater clinical or laboratory manifestations of any level of activity of disease up to grade 4 (see Tables 1 and 2). In the most severe cases the patients were extremely ill with fever of 104° or higher, severe malaise, headache, chest pain, marked rash or arthritis, hematocrit of less than 20, leukopenia of less than 2,000, albuminuria with red cells and white cells and cellular casts. In one of our patients with hypertension, a cerebrovascular accident occurred during an episode of preeclampsia in the ninth month.

The period of pregnancy during which the exacerbation occurred varied greatly, ranging from the first month of pregnancy to 8 weeks after delivery. This is consistent with the more detailed studies by Garsenstein, Pollak, and Kark [84] and Friedman and Rutherford [80], in which similar variation in time of onset of the exacerbation was found, the most common periods being the first 20 weeks and the first 8 weeks postpartum. The majority of the patients in this series in whom exacerbation did not occur remained in constant state with little or no evidence of remission, in contrast to the observations of some others [80, 162]. Many of these patients, however, had rather mild disease at the time of pregnancy. In general, the exacerbations occurred in patients in whom the disease was active at the time of pregnancy or within the few years preceding pregnancy. There was, in our experience, no exacerbation after the patient had been in good clinical remission for 6 to 7 years, as in some series [240] and in contrast to the findings of others [69, 80]. In 2 patients of the series, the initial onset of the disease occurred soon after delivery, 1 by Caesarian section. Pregnancy should be avoided at least during the time the disease is active, as discussed in Chapter 5. Despite the wisdom of preventing pregnancy, use of hormones for contraception may not be advisable. Their use has been followed in a few cases in our experience by increased activity of SLE. Similar observations have been mentioned by Kunkel [139] but there is not adequate knowledge yet to prove a causal relationship.

Therapeutic abortion early in pregnancy was carried out in 2 patients in the present series, and in a few patients not in the series. The activity of the disease was slight at the time of the pregnancies and exacerbation did not follow the abortions. However, the incidence of flares following spontaneous abortion, as reported by others [80, 84, 240], is almost as high as that after full term deliveries, and does not indicate that premature interruption of pregnancy after the first 6 weeks is advisable.

Of great interest is the incidence of toxemia of pregnancy, with preeclampsia in 2 patients of this series during pregnancies occurring after the onset of SLE and also in 1 patient 1 year before the known onset of lupus. Similar or higher incidence was reported by Dubois [69] and Madsen [162]. In 1 of our patients preeclampsia was followed by progression of renal disease, which subsided very gradually over the subsequent 5 years. Death occurred from overwhelming infection. Postmortem examination showed considerable healing of the kidney disease. In the other patient there was very little residual evidence of renal disease. Similarity but not identity of the histologic findings in the kidney in eclampsia and those in SLE has been reported [15, 242] and is of great interest. It raises speculation as to an interrelationship between the two disorders.

Sensitivity to Sunlight and Drugs

Sensitivity to sunlight was present in 34% (48 of 142) in this series and was found to produce some exacerbation of disease either in the skin or systemically. The incidence was the same as that found in the study undertaken to establish criteria for classification of SLE, 37% (91 of 245), and contrasts with that study's finding of only 1% in rheumatoid arthritis (RA) [51]. Despite this relatively frequent exacerbation of SLE by sun exposure, there was no higher incidence of onset of the disease during the summer months, as reported, also, by Dubois [69]. Among the 100 cases in which the month of onset could be determined, the onsets were fairly evenly distributed over the year, 7 or 8 in every month, although there was a slightly higher number in April and in October.

Sensitivity to drugs, usually sulfonamides, was reported in this series in only 20% (28 of 142). However, the reactions to sulfonamides were extremely severe in some cases and led to death in 2 patients, comparable to reports in the literature [52, 111, 141]. Only 6 patients had sensitivity to both sun and drugs. Despite the general fear of reaction to penicillin, our series showed only 1 patient of 54 (2%) with such sensitivity, and similarly few reactions have been reported in other series [69, 146].

Drug Ingestion

Precipitation of a typical clinical and laboratory picture of SLE by drug ingestion, as has been reported by others, has been observed by us in patients not included in the series. The effect of sulfonamides has been discussed. The drugs most commonly found responsible are hydralazine, hydantoin compounds (mephenytoin and diphenylhydantoin), oxazolidine-2-4 dione compounds (tridione), procainamide, and occasionally tetracycline and isoniazid [3, 6, 26, 33, 65, 71, 73, 117, 172, 285]. In 1 patient of this series who had occasional seizures for 3 years before the definite onset of SLE, diphenylhydantoin treatment had been started 9 months before the onset of joint pain and swelling. The disease then progressed steadily, to death in 6 years. It is surely impossible to know whether diphenylhydantoin played any role in the precipitation of the symptoms. In 3 cases seen since the series was closed, it appeared to cause exacerbation with recurrence of rash, fever, and severe leukopenia, all of which subsided after withdrawal of the medication. Procainamide has never produced clinical evidence of renal disease, though the syndrome that may follow its ingestion closely resembles SLE in other respects [33, 71, 172]. Whether or not the patients who present a picture of lupus following drug therapy have the same disease as spontaneously occurring "idiopathic"

SLE cannot be decided on the present knowledge and remains a subject of much discussion [3, 6, 33, 69, 236]. There exist three explanations of the syndrome produced by drugs: 1) that SLE was present before the drug was given and activity was precipitated by the medication; 2) that the syndrome is SLE and is caused by the drug; and 3) that the reaction is not related to SLE. The latter seems somewhat more likely in the case of the incomplete picture caused by procainamide, but the entire question of the nature of drug reactions remain unanswerable at present.

It is of interest that the commonly occurring picture of SLE seen in women in Thailand never includes renal involvement [254]. Investigation has not revealed any drug ingestion that might explain the syndrome.

Clinical Features

Fever

Fever of greater than 100°F orally was found in 61% (87) of the 142 patients. In general it was not above 102° during most of the course, but in the majority of patients it was above 103° at some time, and occasionally as high as 106-107°. Such high temperatures were often seen when acute, severe disease, "lupus crisis," supervened. While associated usually with severe generalized disease, fever of 102° to 105° was not necessarily a forerunner of a rapidly downhill course and in itself is not adequate reason for institution of steroid or immunosuppressive drug therapy, as will be discussed later.

Blood Pressure

Elevation of blood pressure above 150/90 was found at some time in 49% (70) of the 142 patients. Incidence as reported by others varies greatly, usually being less than in this series [57, 69, 102, 103]. In some, the elevation occurred during active disease and disappeared when remission occurred. Only a small percentage had markedly elevated pressures (above 200/120), comparable to the low incidence in other series [11, 106]. In several patients in this series the elevation first appeared during pregnancy. Usually the hypertension persisted indefinitely in such cases, even with clinical remission otherwise, but occasionally it subsided after months or years. In the majority of cases, the hypertension was at least partially responsive to therapy with thiazides, or reserpine, or methyldopa.

Of extreme interest, but hard to explain, is the unusual occurrence of excessively high blood pressure with or without steroids or azathio-prine, such as 250/170, persisting for months and uncontrollable finally by reserpine, thiazides, methyldopa, and diazoxide. Fortu-nately, such a manifestation of the disease is rare [18, 69, 106, 211]. It occurred in 1 patient in our series (aged 17 years) late in the course of the disease, and in 2 women (aged 18 and 40 years) seen since the series was closed. In the first patient, renal failure was not marked. The NPN was 67 mg/100 ml just before death. The glomeruli at post-mortem showed some thickening of the basement membrane and focal areas of crescent formation. Many glomeruli were fibrotic. In one of the latter cases, clinical evidence of glomerulitis was slight: the BUN on the day before death was 17 mg/100 ml and, at autopsy, glomeruli showed no basement membrane changes and only rare hyalinization of afferent arterioles. In the other case, renal function was markedly reduced and the glomeruli showed focal lesions with moderate thick-ening of the basement membrane; an occasional glomerulus showed proliferation of capsule cells and a few were replaced by fibrosis. But the major change in all 3 cases was in the arteries and arterioles. These vessels in the kidneys and elsewhere did show severe vasculitis. In both of the recent cases the clinical course was slowly but steadily downhill, with a cerebrovascular accident due to hemorrhage early in the illness in the first case. Death occurred from terminal pneumonia after 5 to 8 months.

Skin Lesions

Butterfly rash. A characteristic "butterfly" rash was present at some time during the course of the disease in 73% (104) of the 142 patients of this series and a very suspicious but less characteristic rash in butterfly distribution (with fixed erythema, and occasionally scal-ing) in another 8% (11). This incidence is higher than that in many series [11, 57, 119, 220, 267, 271]. Involvement of one cheek or the nose by the typical lesions was considered adequate basis for inclusion as a butterfly rash. Follicular plugging and atrophy often were present in older lesions in the typical cases (79%). In many patients the rash subsided entirely with remission but in many it recurred in exacerba-tion. The presence of a butterfly rash at any time correlated with the system first involved ($p = 0.008$). Twenty-five percent (29) of the 115 patients with butterfly rash had skin involvement, including the face, as the first sign, whereas none of the 27 patients without butterfly rash had skin involvement first. Forty percent (46) of the 115 with butterfly rash had joints involved first, in contrast to 27% (7) of the 27 without rash. There was also a correlation with the occurrence of psychosis, only 15% (17) of the 115 with butterfly rash having psychosis, in contrast to 44% (12) of the 27 without rash ($p = 0.006$).

The presence of abnormal electrophoretic pattern of serum proteins showed some correlation ($p = 0.02$) with the presence of butterfly rash, indicating greater abnormalities in the patients without rash (see Table 4).

Only slight correlation of butterfly rash with age of onset ($p = 0.08$) and number of joints ($p = 0.08$) was found. Sixty percent (69) of the 115 with butterfly rash had onset below the age of 25, in contrast to 40% (11) of the 27 without rash. Involvement of 3 joints or more was observed in 69% (79) of the 115 patients with butterfly rash, in contrast to 82% (22) of the 27 without rash.

No correlation was present between the presence of butterfly rash and joint pain, albuminuria, hematuria, casts, LE cells, or total duration of disease from onset.

Other rash. Rash occurred in other areas of the face or body in 83% (118) of the 142 patients. Only 8% (11) had no rash at any time, a lower incidence than that in other series [11, 57, 69, 102, 103, 220]. The lesions varied markedly even in a single patient, from scattered erythematous macules to typical areas of atrophy, follicular plugging and telangectasia, and rarely to vesicles and ulcerated areas, as described by Keil [127] and Dubois [69].

Histological examination. Histological examination of the skin was obtained by biopsy in 42 patients and at autopsy in 27 others. In 26 (38%) of the 69 the findings were positive for SLE, with hyperkeratinization, epidermal atrophy, liquefaction of the basal layer, and

Table 4. Correlation of abnormal electrophoretic pattern of serum proteins with the presence of butterfly rash ($p = 0.02$). Sixty-nine patients were tested.

| Butterfly rash | Serum globulins | | | |
	a 2 globulin alone elevated	γ globulin alone elevated	both a 2 and γ globulin elevated	Neither a 2 nor γ globulin elevated
Present	19%	26%	20%	33%
Absent	12	50	35	4

homogenization, eosinophilic staining, and fragmentation of collagen. In 7 others the findings were consistent with SLE but not adequate for a definite diagnosis. In 2 patients the changes were consistent with the discoid stage of lupus with more chronic inflammation and fibrosis. Eighteen showed only acute and chronic inflammation of various degrees and 18 were negative. Slight perivascular inflammation was found in 15% (10) of the 69 cases, thickening of the vessel walls in 8% (6) and fibrinoid in the vessel walls in only 4% (3). In one of the latter patients there was severe necrotizing arteritis with associated ulcers.

Pigmentation. Diffuse pigmentation was present in only a few cases of this series, in contrast to the findings of other investigators [11, 69]. Pigmentation localized to areas of skin that had been involved previously was also much less common than that reported in their series.

Fingertip and toe lesions. Fingertip or palmar or toe lesions were present in 35% (50) of the 142 cases, an incidence lower than that reported by Cook [55] in children. The most common lesions were red, often slightly tender areas on palms or fingertips, or diffuse redness of fingertips and occasionally of the entire palm, or telangectasia along the base of nails. Dilated capillaries about the nail were described by Baehr et al. [15]. Similar capillary dilatation along edges of the upper eyelids was fairly common, occuring in 12% (12) of the 97 of the present series for whom information was available. Comparable nail and eyelid telangectasia is seen in dermatomyositis and scleroderma but almost never, if ever, in rheumatoid arthritis, in our experience.

Alopecia. Loss of hair to an excessive degree, usually estimated as 50% or more of the hair, and occasionally with complete alopecia on the scalp, was present in 46% (63) of the 138 patients for whom adequate information was available. Incidence in other series varies markedly. In the series studied for the criteria for classification of SLE [51], the incidence was 43% (105 of 245) as compared to 4% in RA. In other groups it has been somewhat lower [69, 78, 102, 103, 106, 271]. Occasionally the hair loss was the only sign of active disease, but complete loss occurred only with moderately severe disease. Scalp lesions with erythema, scaling, and residual areas of atrophy were associated with the loss in many cases, but considerable loss did take place in the absence of any visible rash on the scalp. In the majority of cases there was complete regrowth of hair, but it was not complete if a significant degree of atrophy was present.

Edema of face. Edema of the face, in the absence of steroid therapy, occurred in 22% (31) of the 142 patients. Ten of these had nephrosis. The most common site was periorbital and the edema was sometimes associated with a reddish or violaceous discoloration, as may be seen in dermatomyositis. Swelling of the eyelids often occurred early in patients with extensive rash in the butterfly distribution but was found also in patients who had no skin rash. In only a few did the edema involve the entire face.

Oral ulcerations. Ulcerations in mouth or on lips were common, occurring in 41% (58) of 141 patients of this series, much more commonly than in many other groups [8, 11, 69, 102, 103]. Mouth lesions ranged from small, red, often tender, slightly elevated lesions, through small vesicles or ulcers, to large vesicular lesions which often ulcerated and usually were very painful. While appearing ordinarily with quite severe disease, they tend to heal slowly and often persist until most of the other signs of activity have disappeared. Usually they finally heal without residual. In general, though not always, the appearance of mouth lesions foretells a fairly severe exacerbation. Whether or not the basis for the lesions is localized areas of vasculitis has not been proved, but it seems likely.

Purpura. Purpura was present at some time in 50% (71) of the 142 patients, a higher incidence than reported in other series [15, 57, 69, 102, 103, 233]. The skin manifestations varied from asymptomatic, pin-point, bright red lesions, to extensive hemorrhagic areas, up to many centimeters in diameter, producing considerable pain. In many cases the purpura was associated with bleeding from the gums. It was usually a manifestation of thrombocytopenia, but in 30% (21) of the 71 cases it occurred in the presence of normal platelet counts and was presumably due to vasculitis. As discussed below, marked hematuria was seen only in patients with either purpura or vasculitis with other manifestations.

Kidneys

Renal involvement is one of the major characteristic features of SLE. In this series 90% (128 of 142) had albuminuria of some degree on at least one occasion and 81% (115) on two occasions or more. In 39% (53) it never exceeded 1 to 2+, but in 51% (73) the albuminuria was 3 to 4+. Of the 90% with albuminuria, approximately one-fifth (26) had urinary tract infection at the time of the examination or within a few months previously, so only 73% (103) of 142 had albuminuria in the absence of infection at any time. However, in 7 of the patients who had urinary tract infection which made the interpretation of the significance of the albuminuria difficult, definite decrease in renal function indicated renal involvement.

Also in 5 of the 15 patients with no albumin in the urine, a significant number of red cells or casts (in two cases cellular casts) were present and, in 2, a decrease in renal function. Therefore, evidence suggestive of renal involvement from urinary and functional studies was present in a total of 86% (122 of 142). This incidence is higher than that reported in some series but corresponds to that in others [11, 18, 57, 109, 159, 255]. The difference presumably results from the use of different criteria in the selection of the series, as discussed above. Possibly inclusion in some series of more patients with a picture closely resembling rheumatoid arthritis, and the use of less strict criteria, explain the variation. Albuminuria was massive in some cases, with excretions up to 17 gm in 24 hours. In many cases, the large excretion of albumin was associated with a clinical picture of nephrosis with edema, and no evidence of renal failure. However, it was not uncommon to find there was associated evidence of glomerulitis and renal failure.

Hematuria. An abnormal number of red cells in the urine (>5 per high-power field in males and >10 in females) was found at least once in 40% (57) of the patients who had no current or recent urinary tract infection. In only 14% (18 patients) were there more than 200 red cells per high-power field at any time and only 12 of these patients had urines in which a high-power field was "loaded with red cells" at any time. Six of the 18 patients had had urinary tract infections. The finding of a relatively infrequent occurrence of large numbers of red cells was somewhat surprising. In 5 of these cases the marked hematuria occurred in association with low platelet counts and purpura, in 10 others in patients who had purpura alone, and in 3 others in patients with decreased platelets. In these cases presumably the hematuria was a reflection of the added effect of thrombocytopenia and/or vasculitis rather than a greater severity of the renal involvement. In fact, 4 of the patients with purpura or decreased platelets and marked hematuria had only minimal other evidence of renal disease. Even of the 10 patients whose urines contained 20 to 200 red cells per high-power field, 5 had purpura, 3 of them having decreased platelet counts. These findings suggest that the glomerulitis of lupus is rarely manifested by marked hematuria in the absence of other cause of capillary bleeding.

Hematuria correlated to some extent with albuminuria without infection ($p = 0.10$). All of 12 patients with over 200 red cells in the urine had albuminuria in the absence of infection. Of 55 patients without an abnormal number of red cells, 81% (45) had albuminuria without infection. Forty-six percent (46) of the 100 patients with albuminuria in the absence of infection had hematuria of some degree in contrast to 19% (3) of the 14 patients with no albumin in the urine.

Hematuria also correlated with the degree of albuminuria ($p = 0.006$). Of the 73 patients with 3 to 4+ albuminuria, including those with infection, 44% (32) had a normal number of red cells in the urine in contrast to 73% (38) of the 53 patients with 1 to 2+ albuminuria. Similarly, 22% (16) of the former group had more than 200 red cells in the urine, in contrast to 5% (3) of the latter group.

In the group of patients with 3 to 4+ albuminuria, marked correlation was found between the presence or absence of hematuria and cellular casts ($p = 0.004$). Forty-eight percent (20) of the 41 patients with abnormal numbers of red cells in the urine and marked albuminuria had cellular casts, in contrast to 13% (4) of the 32 without hematuria. A similar, though less marked, correlation ($p = 0.08$) was noted with the presence of other casts, 53% (22) of the 41 patients with hematuria and marked albuminuria having more than occasional casts in contrast to 32% (10) of the 32 without hematuria. Ten percent (4) of the 41 patients with abnormal numbers of red cells in the urine and marked albuminuria had no casts but 29% (9) of the 32 without hematuria had no casts.

The elevation of NPN or BUN correlated with the presence of hematuria in the group of patients with marked albuminuria ($p = 0.06$). Fifty-six percent (23) of those 41 with hematuria and 3 to 4+ albuminuria had marked elevations of NPN (>50 mg/100 ml) or BUN (>30 mg/100 ml) in contrast to 34% (11) of the 32 without abnormal number of red cells in the urine. Twenty-four percent (10 of 41) of the former group and 51% (16 of 32) of the latter group had no elevation of urea nitrogen.

There was no correlation between the presence of hematuria in patients with marked albuminuria and the presence of edema, duration of disease, course, or severity.

Casts. Casts were present in the urine of 68% (97) of the 142 patients. In 37% (53) only rare or occasional casts were seen. Cellular casts, either of red or white cells, were found in 22% (31) of the patients. Definite red-cell casts were recorded in 7% (10) of the series. In the absence of infection white-cell casts are also suggestive of glomerular disease, as described by others [64, 175].

The presence of casts showed marked correlation with albuminuria in the absence of infection ($p = 0.0001$). Seventy-four percent (74) of the 100 patients with albuminuria without infection had casts in the urine, in contrast to 19% (3) of the 14 with no albumin in the urine. The degree of albuminuria also correlated highly with the presence of casts. Forty-four percent (32) of the 73 patients with 3 to 4+ albuminuria, including those with infection, had casts in the urine (more than rare or occasional) in contrast to only 18% (10) of the 53 with a lesser degree of albuminuria. Eighteen percent (13) of the former group of 73 had no casts, as compared with 36% (19) in the 53 patients with 1 to 2+ albuminuria. Correlation was good also with the presence of cellular casts ($p = 0.006$). Only 9% (5) of the 53 with the smaller amount of albumin in the urine, including those with infection, had cellular casts, in contrast to 31% (23) of the 73 patients with 3 to 4+ albuminuria. Of the 15 patients with no albuminuria, 2 (13%) had cellular casts.

The highest level of NPN or BUN in the serum at any time showed close correlation with the highest degree of albuminuria at any time ($p = <0.001$). Forty-seven percent (34) of the 73 patients with 3 to 4+ albuminuria, including those with infection, had marked elevations of NPN (>50 mg/100 ml) or BUN (>30 mg/100 ml) in contrast to 15% (8) of the 53 with less albuminuria. Seven percent (1) of the 15 with no albuminuria had elevation of NPN or BUN. Similarly, only 35% (26) of the 73 with marked albuminuria had normal urea nitrogen levels at all times, in contrast to 70% (37) of the 53 with 1 to 2+ albuminuria.

Severity of disease correlated slightly with the presence of albuminuria without infection ($p = 0.06$). Thirty-three percent (5) of the 15 patients with no albumin had mild disease with never greater than 2+ severity, in contrast to only 16% (16) of the 100 with albuminuria in the absence of infection. Similarly, only 13% of the patients with 2 or more attacks of grade 3 or greater severity had no albumin, in contrast to 42% who had albuminuria in the absence of infection. In the case of the patients with steadily downhill course to death there was no difference in the percentages that had albuminuria without infection or no albumin in the urine (28 and 25%).

There was no correlation of albuminuria without infection with the presence of cellular casts (in contrast to total number of casts), or edema, or the course of disease, or duration of the disease from onset or from first visit to Massachusetts General Hospital.

Leukocytes. Greater than normal numbers of leukocytes were found in the urine in 58% (82) of the 142 patients, an incidence slightly lower than in some series [18, 187]. Forty percent (57) had between 10 and 100 cells per high-power field but the other 18% (25) had over 100 cells. Of those with increased numbers of leukocytes, only 36% (30) had not had a urinary tract infection. Increased numbers of white cells often appeared in the urine in exacerbation of the renal disease even when numerous cultures under varying conditions disclosed no urinary tract infection, as in other series [69, 187]. In some cases it is an earlier and more impressive abnormality than the usually relatively small number of red cells. As stated above, white-cell casts commonly appear at this time.

Infection. Urinary tract infection was common in this series, cultures being positive at some time in 47% (41) of the 87 patients for whom data were available. The most common organisms were E. coli and Staphylococcus albus. Only occasionally did the urinary tract infection appear to cause exacerbation of the underlying disease, in great contrast to respiratory infections, abscesses, or other infections, which were followed by exacerbations in 85% of the patients. In many of the severe cases infection and exacerbation start almost simultaneously and it is often difficult to determine how much of the clinical picture is due to the infection and how much to active lupus.

Nitrogen retention. Elevation of urea nitrogen in the blood was found at some time in 47% (60) of the 129 patients for whom information was available. This is a much higher incidence that that reported by some investigators [69, 145]. In 16% (20) only moderately increased concentrations were present, between 36 and 50 mg/100 ml, determined as nonprotein nitrogen (NPN), or between 26 and 35 mg, determined as blood urea nitrogen (BUN). In 31% (40) higher concentrations occurred, with NPN values greater than 70 mg/100 ml or BUN greater than 50 mg. The highest NPN not in a terminal episode was 116 mg/100 ml and the highest BUN 198 mg. Elevation of BUN greater than 30 to 38 mg/100 ml is not necessarily an indication that the prognosis is extremely poor or that the patient's life is limited to a few months, as has been stated by some [69, 278]. In fact, 8 patients in our series are living and in fair or good remission 7 to 17 years after exacerbations in which NPN concentrations were above 45 mg/100 ml or BUN concentrations above 30 mg; in 3 of these, NPN values were above 200 mg/100 ml and BUN concentrations were as high as 80 mg.

Renal tubular acidosis. Renal tubular acidosis was noted in 2 of the patients of this series and has been found in a few patients seen since the series ended, similar to the report by Tu and Shearn [270]. In 1 patient, the tubular involvement was limited to marked loss of potassium so severe that 120 meq of potassium orally was required daily to maintain the serum level in the normal range.

Renal Pathology. Kidney biopsies were performed on only 2 of the patients of this series. In one of them, who had severe renal failure at the time of the biopsy and died 8 weeks later, the glomeruli were severely and diffusely damaged. Many nuclear fragments and marked basement membrane thickening were present, and there were mild vascular changes in small arteries and arterioles. In another in whom renal failure was less severe (BUN of 32 mg/100 ml) there were many wire-loop lesions in the biopsied specimen.

Severe, necrotizing arteritis, both acute and chronic, of the inter- and intralobular arcuate vessels, was found in the patient who had removal of one kidney following renal infarction. Death followed renal infarction in the other kidney 3 weeks later, and similar changes were found at autopsy. Perirenal hematoma was found in this kidney, as in a patient described by Dubois [69].

At postmortem the kidneys were enlarged (over 150 gm) in 73% (42) of the 58 patients, the greatest combined weight of the two kidneys being 700 gm in a patient with renal infarction terminally. Glomerulitis with either proliferation or membrane thickening as recognized by light microscopy was noted in 84% (49) of the series of 58, an incidence quite comparable to others [15, 55, 119, 131, 186, 204] but somewhat lower than that found by workers using electron microscopy [18, 47, 53]. In most of the other series, however, either more severe cases were selected or only patients known to have urinary abnormalities were included. Furthermore, of the 11 patients in the present series who showed no glomerular change, 9 were first seen before 1949. Five of these had rapidly downhill courses to death in less than 2 years, and 3 had relatively mild disease for 4 to 17 years and then severe exacerbation with death in less than 2 years. Similarly, the majority (18) of the 26 patients with only very slight glomerular changes were seen before 1949 and 13 of them died within 3 years of the onset of the disease. This suggests that the greater reduction in renal function noted in the patients first seen in 1949 or later may be associated in part at least with duration of disease. Consistent with this thesis is the fact that in 5 of the 6 patients first seen before 1949 who died of renal failure, the duration of disease ranged from 4 to 13 years. In the other it was only 8 months. The increase in severity of renal disease seen after 1950 was noted by Muehrcke et al. [187].

In the present series proliferation was moderate or marked in 40% (23) and slight in 28% (16) of the 58 cases. Hyalinized or fibrosed glomeruli were the only finding in another 5% (3). In 23% (13) the glomerular changes were diffuse and in 51% (30) focal. This may again reflect the high number of the autopsies done on patients first seen before 1949, when less severe renal disease was observed (see Table 10, p. 91). In some of the mild cases only 3 or 4 glomeruli were noted to be abnormal. In all glomeruli that were involved there was some thickening of the basement membrane, as would be expected from the findings of Comerford and Cohen [53], and membrane thickening was the only change in 12% (7). Typical wire loops were seen in 36% (21) of the 58 cases, lower than in other series [15, 55, 95, 131].

Of great interest were the 3 cases (5%) in whom the glomerular lesions had almost completely healed with only fibrosis and hyalinization of the involved glomeruli, as in one woman of 28 who died of septicemia after 6 years of active SLE. The serum level of BUN was 43 mg/100 ml just before death. Clinical evidence of renal disease with a BUN of 30 mg/100 ml had remained quite stationary in the last 3 years of her life. Postmortem examination showed basement membrane thickening and many fibrosed and hyalinized glomeruli.

Tubular and interstitial involvement was present in 43% (25 patients), all but 1 of whom had glomerular changes also. In 36% (21) of the 58 cases, the renal vessels larger than the glomerular capillaries showed inflammation, as found in other series [15, 55, 131, 148, 186]. The changes varied from slight intimal thickening or slight round-cell infiltration to a severe necrotizing process with fibrinoid degeneration and marked infiltration of inflammatory cells in the walls and perivascularly. In 6 cases the changes were indistinguishable from those of periarteritis nodosa. Very marked changes were found also in the 2 patients seen since the series was closed who had excessively high blood pressure (as described above).

Renal infarcts were present in 2 patients, one being septic in a patient with Staphylococcus aureus septicemia. In 1 case there was a massive infarct that led to death. In 4 patients with septicemia there were abscesses, the organisms being Staphylococcus aureus in 2 cases, streptococcus in 1 case, and B. pyocyaneus in the other. A calculus was present in the renal pelvis in 1 patient.

Effect on prognosis. The overall prognosis of the disease varied with the type and severity of renal involvement, as has been noted in all series since the early (1935) report of the severity of the renal lesions by Baehr, Klemperer, and Schifrin [15]. Renal involvement of some degree is present in almost all patients with systemic lupus, whether demonstrated by urinary findings or by light or electron microscopy [18, 53, 187]. In this series of 142 patients albuminuria was present in a total of 90% (128) but only 70% (100) had never had infection. Hematuria of some degree was noted in 40% (57) and casts in 68% (97), cellular in 22% (31). As discussed above, the incidence of clinical abnormalities in other series has varied greatly but in general it has been lower than our finding of probable renal involvement in 86% (122) of the 142 patients in this series. In view of the high incidence of renal involvement, the prognosis in each series reflects the effect of the renal disease. However, if one compares the patients with mild and severe urinary involvement in this series, as based for instance on the degree of albuminuria, the severity varied considerably within each of the two groups.

In general, studies have indicated that there is a moderately good correlation between urinary findings and the degree of damage found by light or electron microscopy [53, 187, 244, 287]. This has been true especially in patients with severe damage.

In other series, the type and degree of involvement seen in biopsies has been compared with duration of disease, and a longer survival has been found in patients showing only glomerulitis, in contrast to those with glomerulonephritis [53, 69, 187, 287]. Opinions vary as to the prognosis when the renal involvement is manifested by the nephrotic syndrome with albuminuria, edema, low serum albumin, relatively normal renal function, normal blood pressure, and no red cells or casts. In our series the prognosis in such patients has usually been good and the course equal to or better than that in patients with mild clinical evidence of glomerulitis, as in some other series [214, 278]. Twenty-nine percent of 44 died in less than 2 years, 27% between 2 and 5 years, 29% between 5 and 10 years, and 13% lived more than 10 years (one lived 35 years). This has been true even when the cholesterol level is high, in contrast to the report by Soffer [244] in which the patients with elevated cholesterol values and nephrosis did not do well.

Despite the apparent serious import of diffuse renal involvement, it is the level and duration of the overall activity of the disease that determines the prognosis. If the patient can heal or greatly lessen the activity of the disease, the renal disease tends to subside even after very severe involvement with extreme failure (see Appendix, cases 1, 2, 3, and 4), and the patients can go into remission for years with varying amounts of reduction in renal function. In our experience such a course has been seen in patients treated with a great variety of agents: aspirin alone in 5 patients; corticosteroids alone in low and high dosage in 7 patients; corticosteroids and azathioprine in 2 patients; azathioprine alone in 1 patient; and, in 1 case, nitrogen mustard. In the latter (case 4), improvement in renal function occurred during four episodes of hospitalization with, on one occasion, the addition of corticosteroid treatment, on another of hydroxychloroquine in addition to the prednisone, on another of azathioprine with the prednisone, and on another, nitrogen mustard. Following this, remission with reduced renal function (BUN 80 mg/100 ml and creatinine 2.0 mg) persisted for 3 years. At the highest degree of failure her BUN was 117 mg per 100 ml and creatinine was 12 mg, with a clearance of 6 liters in 24 hours. After a fifth exacerbation the patient died of renal failure with severe infection associated with a leukocyte count of 1100 per cu mm after treatment with cyclophosphamide, 50 mg per day. In contrast to such remarkable periods of improvement, slow progression of kidney damage may occur during periods of apparent clinical inactivity, similar to the progression of cardiac damage in the course of rheumatic fever in patients with no clinical evidence of activity. Onset of renal failure signifies recurrence or exacerbation of the disease in some cases, comparable to expression of recurrent rheumatic fever activity by the appearance of cardiac failure. The relative importance of the overall disease activity compared with the renal involvement is further manifested by the short duration of life, despite relatively mild renal disease, in the patients seen before 1949 (see Table 10, p. 91). The difficulty in attempting to estimate the prognosis by the degree of renal involvement has been shown in many patients. One example in our series was a girl of 15 in whose record was the statement that "the prognosis here is undoubtedly better in the absence of renal disease." However, activity progressed with central nervous system involvement and recurrent seizures. Death occurred 7 months after the above note was written.

In view of the great variety of conditions of treatment (including hospitalization and medications) that may be associated with healing of the disease and thereby improvement in the renal involvement, the tremendous difficulty in evaluation of the effect of any one therapy is apparent, and it is understandable why such differences of opinion exist as to the effect of various medications. The details of therapy and the relatively unsuccessful attempts to do controlled studies of the effects of various therapies will be discussed later. At this time, emphasis should be placed on the necessity for treating the patient to produce a lessening in the disease activity, rather than attempting to consider the renal disease as a separate event, requiring special treatment, as is usually done by most investigators.

Joints

Joint involvement as manifested by pain was present in 91% (129) of the 142 patients. As noted above, this high percentage may be in part related to the fact that this series was seen by physicians treating especially patients with rheumatic disease, but the incidence in many other series is comparable [11, 57, 69, 103, 106, 119, 159, 173, 216, 267]. Joint involvement was intermittent in 64% (83) of the 129 patients on whom information was available. Such high incidence is comparable with that reported by Armas-Cruz [11]. It is higher than the incidence of intermittent arthritis in most series of patients with rheumatoid arthritis and represents a very characteristic finding in lupus. The individual attacks may last a few hours to several days or even 3 to 4 weeks, then subside, and recur at greatly varying intervals, from a day or two to weeks or months. Morning stiffness with significant increase in stiffness and usually in pain in the morning was described by 73% (51) of the 71 patients on whom information was available. This incidence is slightly greater than that reported by Dubois [69] and Labowitz and Schumacher [144], and probably as high as the usual occurrence in rheumatoid arthritis, 75% [56].

In 12% (17) of the 142 patients, fewer than three joints were involved objectively by swelling, effusion, pain, or tenderness, with 74% (105) having signs in three joints or more. Only 14% (20) had no objective involvement at any time. Swelling of one or more joints was noted in 74% (105) of the series.

Deforming arthritis. Chronic joint involvement with deformity developed in 30% (43) of the 142 patients, comparable to the findings in other series [11, 69, 103, 149]. In many cases only a few joints were involved, deformities being limited to a few phalangeal joints, but in a small number of patients severe, generalized, crippling deformities were present. "Swan neck" deformities were found in 10 cases. Joints with such involvement were absolutely indistinguishable clinically from those of severe rheumatoid arthritis. Chronic involvement occurred most commonly in the metacarpophalangeal and proximal interphalangeal joints. X-rays of joints were obtained in 72 patients, and 40% (29) showed some degree of atrophy around the joints consistent with the histological findings of Cruickshank [61]. In 2 cases with chronic involvement x-rays showed very little or no change, similar to the findings in some other series [69, 144, 193]. Only 6 had definite erosions, due in 2 cases to aseptic necrosis.

Aseptic necrosis. Only 2 patients in this series developed aseptic necrosis, a lower incidence than in other series [69, 144], possibly because of the smaller number of patients treated with steroids. Two other patients with aseptic necrosis have been seen since the series was closed. While reported occasionally in patients with lupus who have not been treated with steroids, it usually occurs after steroid therapy [155, 219, 241]. One of the patients in this series had had steroids on five occasions over 10 years for periods ranging from 2 to 12 months, but never greater dosage than 40 mg of prednisone and usually less than 20 mg. The other patient had never taken steroids. In addition to the relatively common involvement of hips, the first patient had also similar changes in the 4th and 5th lumbar vertebrae. Such localization has not been reported previously. Fortunately, in contrast to the usual progression, the femoral heads remained relatively normal in shape for 3 years and there were no clinical signs until 3 years later.

Synovial biopsy. Two synovial biopsies showed chronic, nonspecific synovitis. One other was negative. A biopsy from the Achilles tendon, which had ruptured, showed tenosynovitis with abundant vascularization and granulation tissue. Synovitis of some degree was present in 35% (13) of the 38 patients in whom joints were examined at postmortem, a slightly lower incidence than that found by Labowitz and Schumacher [144] and Cruickshank [61]. In 3 cases there was only slight proliferation of the synovial cells. Mild diffuse infiltration with lymphocytes and plasma cells was present in 6 patients and focal areas in 1 other. Some edema was present in 3 cases. Eight had areas of fibrinoid necrosis, in 1 case occurring throughout the entire depth of the synovial tissue as well as superficially, similar to the findings in joints [144] and also in tendon sheaths by Cruickshank [61]. Fluid ranging in volume from 8 to 100 ml was found in 7 cases, and was noted to be viscous in 5. This correlates with the high viscosity found clinically in effusions in SLE. In some cases an unusual degree of hyaline material was observed just below the synovial surface. It is intriguing to speculate as to whether this is related to the high concentration of mucin and the high viscosity found in synovial fluids in lupus, findings which indicate a high degree of polymerization of hyaluronic acid despite the inflammation, in great contrast to the usual findings in rheumatoid arthritis. Of interest in this respect is the fact that the pericardium had a mucoid appearance in 3 patients, the peritoneal fluid in 5 cases, and in 3 other patients, fatty areas had a mucinous ground substance. Asboe-Hansen [13] reported an increase in the amount of "hyaluronic acid" in the corium in patients with SLE.

Destruction of cartilage or bone was relatively rare (3%) (4 of 142 patients). Superimposed infectious arthritis was present in only 1 patient in this series of autopsies. A higher incidence might have been expected from the apparent increased permeability to bacteria present in inflamed joints, as is seen not uncommonly in rheumatoid arthritis [210]. Infectious arthritis was seen clinically in this series in 3 patients, in 1 due to E. coli and in 2 to Staphylococcus aureus. All responded well to antibiotic therapy. Involvement of vessels was present in the synovial tissues in 10 patients, an incidence slightly lower than that in other series [61, 144, 158], usually with proliferation of the intima and slight infiltration of lymphocytes and mononuclears in the walls.

Spondylitis. Spondylitis was present in only 1 of the 142 patients. Motions of lumbar and dorsal spine were markedly limited. There was pain and stiffness throughout, and chest expansion was only 0.5 inch, but x-rays were negative. It is of interest that this patient was the only one who had definite aortic insufficiency, though two others had aortic diastolic murmurs.

Tendon rupture. Rupture of the Achilles tendon occurred in 2 patients and rupture of the patellar tendon on a separate occasion in 1 of these patients. This represents an incidence of tendon rupture comparable to that reported by others [168, 273]. They also noted rupture of the patellar as well as the Achilles tendons. In all cases the patients were receiving steroids.

Chest Pain

Chest pain occurred commonly and often persisted after all other symptoms had subsided. It was present in 78% (75) of the 97 patients on whom information was available, an incidence higher than that found by Hejtmancik et al. [106]. Often when a rub was not present it was difficult to differentiate pleural from skeletal pain. The latter occurred most commonly in the lower chest anteriorly on either side and was usually associated with tenderness along the ribs or costochondral or sternocostal junctions. In 29% (28) of the 97 patients who had chest pain it was only pleural in origin, and in 33% (32) skeletal only, insofar as could be determined. In another 37% (35) both pleural and skeletal pain were present. Anginal pain was present in 3 patients and probable angina occurred in 5 others. The skeletal pain over lower ribs anteriorly or in axillae is quite characteristic of lupus and persists longer than many other symptoms, as noted by Haserick [103]. Even more characteristic is its recurrence with mild flare of disease activity, often as the only clinical manifestation or occasionally in association with fatigue or other mild symptoms.

Abdominal Pain

Abdominal pain is very common in lupus; in our series it occurred in 62% (61) of the 99 patients on whom information was available. This incidence is much higher than in other reports [69, 102, 103]. It may be extremely severe, especially when associated with a lupus "crisis." In many cases with severe pain, whether due to peritonitis or vasculitis in organs, it is extremely difficult to determine whether there is any condition which requires surgical intervention such as appendicitis or ruptured viscus [27, 140, 200, 203]. This is especially true when the patient is receiving large doses of steroids with their alteration of physical findings, especially spasm and rebound tenderness. In this difficult situation, frequent observation, often hourly, by both medical and surgical physicians is necessary, as will be discussed under treatment.

Ascites

Ascites was present in 6 patients who were not receiving steroids and in 5 others who were on steroid therapy, a total incidence of 8% (11 of 142). In some series a slightly higher incidence has been reported [11, 57, 69]. Peritoneal involvement was present at postmortem examination in 63% (37 of 58 cases). The incidence in other series has varied greatly [55, 119, 186]. The volume of fluid varied from less than 10 ml to 4,000 ml. Adhesions were found most commonly over spleen and liver, but occurred over the stomach, intestines, pelvic organs, and various parts of the abdominal wall. They varied from thin fibrinous and fibrous strands to firm, old adhesions, and to large areas of complete adhesion, usually between the liver and the diaphragm. In 5 cases the peritoneal fluid was mucinous. Marked fibrinoid degeneration was present in 1 patient. The mesentery in 1 case showed numerous small foci of hemorrhage, necrosis, and infiltration of neutrophils.

Gastrointestinal Tract

Dysphagia of moderate degree was present in only 5 of the patients but mild difficulty or pain on swallowing occurred in 17 others. The incidence of dysphagia is similar to that reported by others [15, 69, 102]. Barium swallow, performed in 42 of the patients of the present series, revealed abnormalities in 4. The usual changes were slightly reduced peristalsis and slight dilatation of the lower esophagus, as found by Tatelman and Keech [264]. In 1 patient there was slight narrowing with partial obstruction at the lower end of the esophagus with dilatation and diminished peristalsis. The obstruction was relieved after esophagoscopy.

Acute esophagitis with fibrinoid necrosis, diffuse inflammatory infiltrate, and edema was present at postmortem examination in 3 cases. In another, gelatinous material surrounded the esophagus, and in still another, unusually fibrotic areolar tissue bound the esophagus to adjacent structures. In 1 patient acute and chronic inflammation of the tongue was found. Severe ulceration of the pyriform sinuses was present in 1 case with fibrinoid necrosis, infiltration of polymorphonuclears, blood vessel proliferation and hemorrhage. The ulcerations extended between the hyoid bone and the laryngeal cartilage.

Peptic ulceration was apparent clinically in only 7 of the 35 patients in whom x-ray studies were performed. Five of these 7 were receiving steroids. Gastrointestinal ulcerations were present in 21% (12) of the 58 cases at postmortem, occurring in the esophagus, stomach, or duodenum in 10% (6). All but one of the latter patients were being treated with steroids and it was impossible to determine whether the peptic ulcerations were related to the disease or to the treatment. However, it seems probable that the intestinal ulcerations were due to active lupus. In 1 case a severe ulcerative process extended from the last 30 cm of the terminal ileum through the entire colon and rectum. Complete disappearance of the mucosa of the colon, with partial necrosis, congestion and hemorrhage, occurred in another patient who was uremic. In this case it was impossible to determine whether the colitis was due to lupus or to uremia or both.

Muscle

Muscle involvement as manifested by pain and tenderness of muscles and some weakness was common, and extreme weakness occurred in 15% (21 of the 142 patients). In most of these patients marked atrophy of muscles was present. In the severe cases the clinical picture was that of complete paralysis of the affected extremities with flaccid muscles and absent reflexes. Enzyme levels were not determined in enough patients to know the incidence of abnormal values but elevation of creatine phosphokinase up to 500 units occurred. In patients seen recently, levels of 900 units have been found. In many cases the marked elevation of serum glutamic oxalic transaminase or lactic acid dehydrogenase was apparently due, in part at least, to muscle involvement. With subsidence of the disease complete recovery of muscle strength usually occurred. Occasionally localized weakness persisted, and not uncommonly there was some residual atrophy.

Muscle biopsies were performed in 15 patients. Seven were entirely negative but 5 showed lymphocytic and plasma cell infiltration perivascularly, 2 showed chronic myositis and fibrositis, and 1 was entirely consistent with dermatomyositis. The incidence of abnormalities was greater (53%) (75 of 142 cases) than that found at postmortem (24%) (14 of 58 cases). The more frequent demonstration of changes by biopsy was presumably due to the opportunity to choose the obviously involved muscles. At postmortem the incidence of inflammatory foci in muscles was comparable to that reported by Klemperer et al. [131]. Since they were noted on examination of routine samples of muscle without extensive search, it is probable that the actual incidence of such foci in muscles is much higher. The lesions consisted of perivascular infiltration of lymphocytes, plasma cells, and monocytes, and occasionally neutrophils and macrophages. In 2 cases there was increased interstitial connective tissue. Hyalinization and atrophy of some fibers was noted in 6 patients and severely damaged fibers in 1. A few vessels showed medial degeneration in 1 case.

Neurological and Psychological Involvement

Diplopia. An unexpected frequency of diplopia or a complaint of considerable blurring of vision was found in this series, being present in 26% (34 of 142), a much higher incidence than in other reports [48, 69, 103]. In the majority of cases it was not possible to determine whether the symptoms were due to slight muscle weakness or to nerve involvement. In a few cases in which the diplopia was marked with obvious deviation of eyes on movements in one direction or another (as for instance, with right lateral upward gaze), it was apparent that there was nerve involvement, presumably from localized vasculitis. In one patient, for instance, there was "right internuclear ophthalmoplegia." Intermittent ophthalmoplegia with horizontal mystagmus of the abducting eye on lateral gaze was present in another.

Psychoses. Psychoses of different degrees occurred in 28% (40) of the 142 patients, an incidence similar to that reported in other series [69, 102, 109, 159, 216]. The clinical pictures were varied but included 29 with depressions, 1 with resultant suicide while on steroid therapy. Associated with the depression was paranoia in 4 patients and confusion in 4. Five patients had hysteria, slight in 3 of them. Headache and memory loss were common. In a few patients, extreme withdrawal and refusal to talk or eat or move occurred. Catatonia was present in 2 patients. All aspects of "senile brain disease" were noted in one woman of 52. The psychoses usually persisted for weeks or months and in 1 case for over a year. Similar manifestations have been reported by many [22, 48, 62, 165, 274].

Seventy-four percent of the psychotic episodes appeared when the patients were not receiving steroids. In other cases, it was often not possible to tell whether the psychosis was a manifestation of the disease, or caused by the steroid therapy or due to a combination of the two factors. In only 1 case in which the dose of steroids was increased because of the appearance of the psychosis was there any apparent improvement in the symptoms. In several cases, despite the fact that steroid dosage was reduced steadily, the psychosis improved, but it was impossible to determine whether there was any interrelationship.

The occurrence of a lesser amount of active renal disease in the patients with psychosis is comparable to the observations of Clark and Bailey [48] and Cheatum et al. [47] of very little active renal disease in their patients with central nervous system involvement. In our series only 50% of the 40 patients with psychosis had any urinary evidence of active nephritis.

Convulsions. Convulsions were slightly less common than in some other series [48, 69, 102, 103, 221]. Some patients had recurrence of seizures in rapid succession but the majority had only a single seizure at any one time. They occurred in 11% (7) of the 60 patients seen since 1949 at some stage of their disease not in a terminal episode, and in another 6% (4) terminally. In the 82 patients seen before 1949, the same percentage had seizures but 70% (10 of 14) occurred terminally. They were the apparent immediate cause of death in several patients. A few never regained consciousness; others had severe respiratory distress and anoxia after the seizure despite oxygen therapy and died within a few hours. Apparently the patients could not withstand the stress of the seizure in the presence of extremely active disease. How much of the difficulty was associated with anoxia was not determined, but the marked anoxia subsequent to the seizure in many cases has indicated the advisability of having oxygen therapy available for very sick patients for immediate use if seizures occur, as is discussed in Chapter 5. It is of interest that 1 patient had occasional seizures for 3 years before the accepted onset of SLE.

Psychoses and seizures usually did not occur in the same patient. In only 15% of the patients with either manifestation did the other appear at any time.

In 6 cases with severe hypertension, cerebral hemorrhage with resulting hemiparesis occurred and in 1 case with thrombocytopenia. In 1 patient with circulating anticoagulant a fatal hemorrhage from a ruptured saccular aneurysm of the right internal carotid posterior communicating artery occurred 5 years after the series was closed. In such patients the resulting paralysis persisted if the patient lived, in contrast to the relatively rapid subsidence, in days or weeks, of complete hemiplegia or paresis following cerebral vascular accidents in many lupus patients. These occurred in 5 patients without hypertension greater than 150/95 or thrombocytopenia. Nine other patients had abnormal plantar or Hoffman reflexes, clonus and sensory changes. It is probable, as indicated by Johnson and Richardson [121] and Dubois [69], that such accidents were secondary to vasculitis without gross hemorrhage and apparently subsided with decrease in spasm. There is little evidence of any effect of therapy, as will be discussed later (see Chapter 5). One of the characteristics of the neurological abnormalities in this disease is the rapid rate of change that may occur.

Only 1 patient had paraplegia, associated with severe psychosis. Autopsy showed remarkable degeneration of the white matter of the entire spinal cord and multiple microinfarcts, as described in detail by

Johnson and Richardson [121]. The probability that these changes resulted from arteritis similar to that described by Dubois [69] is intriguing.

Chorea. Two patients had chorea with persistent involuntary movements. It has been reported occasionally by other investigators [42, 48, 86, 117, 146, 196, 218]. Postmortem examination in 1 showed numerous microinfarcts and several small arteries filled with necrotic material. Athetoid movements were present in 2 patients.

Peripheral neuropathy of slight degree was not uncommon but severe neuropathy was present in only 6 patients, an incidence slightly higher than that in other series [48, 69, 102, 103]. Individual cases have been reported by others [107, 152, 223].

Facial palsy occurred in only 1 patient, but weakness of facial muscles in 2 others.

All neurological abnormalities in SLE may change rapidly, as noted above. Within the span of 24 hours, examination may show the appearance and disappearance of diplopia and abnormalities of extraocular movements; short periods of localized hypesthesia; presence and then absence of clonus; alteration in a few hours in plantar reflexes; varying degrees of paresis in extremities, changing in a few hours; and tremor of extremities or tongue of varying duration. Again it seems probable that such signs are secondary to vasculitis, and change with variations in associated spasm.

Electroencephalograms. Electroencephalograms were obtained in 16 patients. Three were entirely normal and 2 others only questionably abnormal. Four showed generalized or irregular slight slowing. Four manifested moderate diffuse abnormality. In 3 others the changes were entirely consistent with epilepsy. Two of these patients had subsequent seizures and the other had had seizures for 3 years before the definitive onset of her disease. The incidence of abnormalities was approximately the same as in other series [69, 151, 221].

Electromyogram was performed in only 1 patient and was consistent with peripheral neuropathy.

Examination of the brain at postmortem was negative in 13 patients (35% of 37). Brain infarct or definite nerve cell loss was found in 36% of the 37 patients examined. Other abnormalities were found in 38% of the cases. Nineteen of the 37 cases are the same as those included in the detailed study of 24 cases by Johnson and Richardson [121]. Infarcts ranged from single small areas in many cases to multiple infarctions in 1 patient, involving cortex, brain stem, and cerebellum. Areas

of loss of nerve cells were small and scattered in 11 patients, but widespread or diffuse in the other 5. In 1 patient with acute mastoiditis and
meningitis there was a septic infarct in the right cerebellar lobe. Old
infarcts in the basal ganglia were present in two cases. In most of the
areas of loss of cells there was increase in the number of astrocytes and
microglial proliferation. A similar reaction was present in 7 other
cases in which nerve cell loss was not apparent.

Massive fresh intracerebral hemorrhage was present in 5 patients.
Extensive subarachnoid hemorrhage was found in 1 of the patients
who died after the series was ended. It resulted from rupture of a saccular aneurysm of the right internal carotid posterior communicating
artery. Small fresh hemorrhages were noted in 3 patients. Moderate
thickening or cloudiness of the pia-arachnoid was found in 8 cases.
Subarachnoid inflammatory exudate was present in 4 patients, 1 of
whom had cryptococcosis. Cerebral vessels showed severe necrotizing
vasculitis in 4 cases with endothelial proliferation, hyalinization and
fibrinoid necrosis of the walls, and infiltration of plasma cells, lymphocytes, macrophages, and occasional neutrophils in the adventitia,
and occasional fibrin perivascularly. The vasculitis was similar to that
reported by Baš and Vachtenheim [21]. In 7 other cases there were
similar, less severe changes. The vessels involved were usually small
arteries or arterioles, as discussed by Johnson and Richardson [121].
In 1 patient capillaries in the cord were also involved. Some arteries in
3 patients were filled with eosinophilic material. Minimal atherosclerosis of cerebral vessels was the only abnormality in 3 patients. Slight
enlargement of the fissures was present in 2 cases, and moderate dilatation of the cerebral ventricles in 1.

The relatively good correlation of the presence of microinfarcts and
presumably causative vascular abnormalities with the clinical signs in
most of the 19 cases of this series studied by Johnson and Richardson
has been discussed in detail by them [121]. There was, however, little
or no correlation of the site of damage with the clinical findings. In the
additional 18 patients of this series in whom the brains were examined
at autopsy there was, by chance, a much lower incidence of neurological or psychological abnormalities. Seizures occurred in only 3 patients (17%) in contrast to 54% in their series of 24; abnormalities of
cranial nerve function in 22% in contrast to 41%; hemiparesis in 6%
in contrast to 12%; chorea in 6% in contrast to zero; psychoses in
22% in contrast to 33%.

Twelve patients in the total of 37 in our series in whom the brains were examined had seizures. At autopsy 7 showed microinfarcts or diffuse nerve cell loss; 2 had microhemorrhages; 2 had large intracerebral hemorrhages; 5 showed vasculitis in small vessels, 3 with necrosis of parts of the walls; and 2 were negative except for moderate engorgement of the small vessels in 1. Pathologic changes in the patient with chorea were numerous microinfarcts and several small arteries filled with necrotic material. In the 11 patients with psychoses, postmortem examination showed 7 with microinfarcts; 1 with a large cerebral hemorrhage; 4 with vasculitis; 2 with minimal changes—slight thickening of meninges in 1 and moderate engorgement of small vessels in the other; and 1 negative. It is interesting to speculate as to whether the small size of infarcts may correlate with the transient nature of the clinical signs.

Eye

Involvement of the eye is not common. Cytoid bodies were seen in this series in 8 of 97 patients. They tended to disappear as the activity of the disease subsided. The incidence is similar to that found by Cohen et al. [51] in the study to formulate criteria for classification of patients with SLE (8%), 20 of 245. They found no cytoid bodies in RA in that study. The incidence was slightly higher in other series of SLE [169, 246, 267]. Papilledema, occasionally with hemorrhages and exudates, has been reported by several investigators [32, 169, 230]. Blindness has occurred rarely [32, 230].

Subcutaneous Nodules

Subcutaneous nodules were found at some time on examination in a surprisingly high percentage (22%, 31) of the 140 patients on whom information was available, in contrast to smaller percentages (5 to 10%) found in most other series [69, 102, 103, 267]. They tended to be relatively small (about 5 mm in diameter), compared to the average size of similar nodules in rheumatoid arthritis, and were often of short duration. Of interest was the finding that nodules were not present in the 12 patients who had no joint pain ($p = 0.15$) nor in the 18 patients who had no objective joint signs ($p = 0.01$). The incidence of nodules showed no relationship to the presence of butterfly rash, LE cells, rheumatoid factor, or elevated serum globulin levels. In patients first seen since 1949 there was no correlation between the presence of nodules and the course, severity, or duration of the disease or the number of patients in the series who died.

At postmortem examination subcutaneous nodules were found in only 3% (2) of the 58 patients, in contrast to the rather high percentage (22%, 31 of 140) in whom nodules were found at some time during the course of the disease. In one nodule at postmortem examination there was a mild chronic inflammatory reaction in the corium and shredded collagen and fibrinoid parallel to the surface. In the 5 biopsies performed the histological pictures varied from diffuse granulomatous tissue to foci of fibrinoid principally about vessels, or to extensive fibrinoid degeneration. In no case was there the characteristic organization of typical rheumatoid nodules with a center of fibrinoid and often necrotic debris, a rim of proliferating mesenchymal cells in palisade formation, and a surrounding zone of infiltrating cells, largely mononuclear. However, in 1 case, indication of such organization was seen but there was no palisade formation. The lack of the typical features of rheumatoid nodules is similar to the report of Larson [146] but in great contrast to the 6 cases reported by Hahn, Yardley and Stevens [99]. In the 3 of their cases which were biopsied the nodules were indistinguishable from those of rheumatoid arthritis.

Lymphadenopathy

Palpable lymph nodes in areas other than the anterior cervical region were found in 78% of the patients, a higher incidence than that in other series [69, 102, 103, 119]. Those in the posterior cervical region were usually small (<5 mm) but in both cervical and axillary areas the nodes were occasionally as large as 1 to 2 cm. Commonly, lymph node enlargement persisted after the majority of other signs had subsided, and frequently recurred early in exacerbations. In a few cases lymph nodes remained enlarged after the disease had been in apparent remission for many years. Lymph node biopsies showed hyperplasia in 7 cases, 1 of which was called giant follicular lymphoma in an outside hospital, chronic lymphadenitis in 6, and only 1 of 14 was normal. In 1 of those with lymphadenitis, most of the inflammatory cells were eosinophils.

At postmortem examination lymph nodes, including retroperitoneal, hilar, and axillary, were enlarged in 78% (45) of the 58 patients, in accord with the high incidence of lymphadenopathy (78%) found clinically and in other series [95, 186]. Distortion of the architecture by engorgement of the sinuses and infiltration with many plasma cells, monocytes, polymorphonuclears, and macrophages was found in 35% (20 of 58). These changes are quite characteristic of SLE.

In 2 cases the architecture was obliterated by masses of granular necrosis comparable to the findings of Klemperer et al [131]. In 6 other cases there was moderate to marked necrosis with surrounding granulomatous tissue and infiltration of polymorphonuclears, monocytes, plasma cells, and phagocytes. The follicles were obliterated in 10 cases. Germinal centers were absent in 5 patients, atrophic in 2, and infiltrated with lymphocytes and monocytes in 1. Reticular hyperplasia was marked in 6 cases. Fibrinoid necrosis was noted in 4 patients and hematoxylin bodies in 1. Marked phagocytosis of erythrocytes was found in 2 cases. Four mesenteric glands were calcified. New growth of capillaries throughout was noted in 5 patients, "onion skin" thickening of arterioles in 2, and thrombosis of small vessels with perivascular fibrosis and inflammation in 2. In 1 case the mediastinal nodes showed a rather extensive granulomatous response with central necrosis, epithelioid cells, and Langhans' giant cells, suggesting tuberculosis. No acid-fast organisms were seen.

Thymus

No abnormality of the thymus was recognized clinically. At postmortem 1 showed hyperplasia, 32 were negative and 26 not identified. Thymectomy was not performed on any of these patients but lack of beneficial effect following this procedure has been reported by others [5, 161, 164, 180].

Thyroid

Enlargement of the thyroid was found in 15% (15) of the 97 patients on whom adequate information was available. In general, the thyroid was not markedly enlarged, being 1½ to 2 times the normal size. Myxedema was present in one of the patients with enlarged thyroid and hyperthyroidism in another, but the majority were euthyroid. Hijmans et al. [108] observed 5 patients with SLE and Hashimoto's thyroiditis. However, in a study of 74 matched, autopsy-proven cases of Hashimoto's disease there was no increase in the incidence of rheumatic disease, though in a clinical study there was suggestive increase of SLE and RA in the group with thyroiditis. Biopsies were performed on only 3 patients of our series but the results were characteristic of thyroiditis. In only a few of the patients of this series were antithyroglobulin antibodies determined. The results ranged from 1:80 to 1:1019. One patient had had a thyroid adenoma removed 6 years before the known onset of SLE.

At postmortem examination the thyroid showed abnormalities, usually slight, in only 7 patients. One had acute and chronic thyroiditis with infiltration of lymphocytes and plasma cells, fibroblastic proliferation, and focal fibrinoid necrosis. In 1 case there was infiltration of the capsule with polymorphonuclears and, in another, perifollicular lymphocytic infiltration. Small abscesses, due to Staphylococcus aureus, were present in 2 patients. A small colloid adenoma was noted in 1 case and a few calculi in another.

Heart

Cardiac involvement of some type was common. In 56% (74) of the 133 chest x-rays enlargement of the heart was found, a much higher incidence than in other series [69, 102, 103, 106]. As stated below, pericardial effusion was thought to be present in less than one-third of these.

Pericardium. Pericardial rub was heard in 29% (41) of the 142 patients, in great contrast to the infrequent occurrence in patients with rheumatoid arthritis (2%) [146, 277] and in higher incidence than in other series [69, 106, 232]. A detectable amount of pericardial fluid in patients with lupus is less common than a rub, being noted clinically in only 17% (23 of 133) in this series. Despite the frequent occurrence of pericarditis, tamponade is uncommon, being reported in only a few cases [38, 103, 117, 135, 224]. Tamponade was present in only 1 patient of this series and suspected in 1 other. Pericardectomy was performed in the former, but cardiac arrest occurred during the operation. Occurrence of pericardial rub or appearance of effusion is not necessarily a cause for great concern or an indication for more vigorous therapy such as steroids (see discussion in Chapter 5). Careful watching is essential but in the great majority of cases no physiological impairment supervenes and the pericarditis subsides with remission of the acute attack. It does not necessarily signify a poor prognosis, as recognized also by Hejtmancik et al. [106].

The presence of pericarditis, often in addition to myocarditis, presumably explains the very common occurrence of abnormal T waves in the electrocardiogram, as found in 75% (80) of the 107 patients of this series in whom the test was done, a figure comparable to that in other series [38, 106]. In 23% (25) the abnormality was only slightly beyond the limits of normal, but in the other 52% the changes were definitely abnormal, being very marked in some cases. Frequently the T waves returned to normal as the disease activity subsided.

At postmortem, pericardial involvement was found in 83% (48 of 58), an incidence similar to that in some series [69, 92, 114] though higher than in most other series [15, 38, 55, 90, 93, 119, 146, 186], and in the series of children reported by Brigden et al. [38]. Pericarditis at postmortem in rheumatoid arthritis has been reported to occur in 25% to 50% of the cases [147, 245, 282]. Fluid present in 40% (23) of 58 patients varied in volume from 10 to 700 ml. It was hemorrhagic in only 2 cases, 1 after aspiration before death. Tamponade is very rare, as stated above. Microscopic inflammatory changes present in 34% (20 of 58 cases) showed great variation in type and degree. Several had only rare foci of fibrinoid degeneration or minimal infiltration of inflammatory cells. In others, extensive areas of fibrinoid degeneration and/or heavy infiltration of lymphocytes, plasma cells, monocytes, and occassionally neutrophils or large histiocytes were present. In a few cases there was marked edema or hemorrhagic areas and, in 3 patients, mucoid material occurred. A superficial layer of fibrin was occasionally present. Vessels in the pericardium in 10 cases showed inflammatory changes of varying degrees with proliferation of the intima, occasional areas of fibrinoid degeneration, and perivascular infiltration of inflammatory cells. In 1 case there were numerous hematoxylin bodies. Adhesions ranged from fibrous and fibrinous strands in 16% (9 of 58 cases) to large areas of adhesion with complete obliteration of the pericardial sac in 25% (15). Complete chronic adhesive pericarditis was not seen but has been reported [106, 283]. In one case the epicardium of the right ventricle contained several 2-cm calcified nodules.

Myocardium. Myocardial involvement is less common. Indication of it was given by the 10% (13) of the 128 patients tested in whom the P-R interval was prolonged (>0.20 with a rate of 100 or >0.18 with a rate of 120). It presumably played a role in the EKG changes discussed above. A gallop was present in 25% (36) of the 142 patients at some time, an incidence to be compared with reported variations from 12 to 50% [11, 135, 233]. Complete atrioventricular dissociation was present in 1 case reported by Moffitt [182].

Cardiac involvement, in addition to pericarditis, was found frequently at postmortem examination. Myocarditis, varying from small areas of perivascular inflammtion to more widespread diffuse interstitial inflammation occurred in 42% (22 of 58 cases), comparable to other series [55, 114, 131, 135, 146, 186]. Fibrinoid degeneration was present in 9 cases. Typical Aschoff nodules were seen in 2 patients. In

2 cases abscesses were associated with Staphylococcus aureus septice-mia. The relatively mild changes in the majority of cases are consistent with the minimal evidence of myocarditis usually present clinically.

Myocardial infarction was recognized clinically in 3 patients, 1 woman aged 26, 1 aged 48, and 1 aged 51. In another patient of 27, in whom postmortem examination showed a small healing infarct, an-gina had been present for 2 to 3 months before death. In all cases the infarction occurred when activity of lupus was marked. The symp-toms and signs in the first 3 patients were entirely characteristic of myocardial infarction. In 1 case extreme ventricular irritability was present.

In 2 cases at postmortem old myocardial infarctions were present, one in a patient of 27 years, known to have had a severe infarction 1 year before death, and the other in a patient of 48 years who had had one infarct years before death and another terminally. Of great inter-est is the question as to whether the infarctions resulted from vasculitis or atherosclerosis of the coronary vessels. In the patient who died 1 year after the myocardial infarction, postmortem examination dis-closed severe atherosclerosis of the involved vessel, the anterior de-scending artery, but one section of the vessel adjacent to the old thrombus showed acute inflammation and necrosis in both intima and muscularis, and one focus of hemorrhage and acute inflammation in the adventitia. The possibility that vasculitis played a role in the in-farction cannot be ruled out. In cases reported by others [55, 69, 106, 265] coronary arteritis was found. In the second case, there was mod-erate atherosclerosis and no definite evidence of vasculitis.

A third patient of 27 years had a small healing infarct. Thirteen others had areas of fibrosis of varying size, often scattered diffusely throughout the heart, replacing muscle cells. Edema was marked in 3 cases. Vessels in the heart, other than the coronary arteries described above, showed varying degrees of intimal proliferation, with occa-sional areas of fibrinoid degeneration and infiltrate of inflammatory cells, usually in the adventitia, in 8 patients. Slight to moderate ather-osclerosis was present in 2 others, not associated with infarcts.

Valves. Clinical evidence of valvulitis was not common. Systolic murmurs of greater than grade 2 out of 4 intensity and thought to be organic in origin occurred in 16% (23) of the 142 patients, a somewhat lower incidence than that reported in other series [69, 102, 103, 106, 232]. In only 3 patients was an aortic diastolic murmur present at any time, but one has been noted in 4 patients seen since the series was closed. It is of great interest, but not yet explainable, that at least two of the three instances of aortic insufficiency reported by Shulman and Christian [235] occurred in patients with SLE which was clinically atypical and very suggestive of rheumatoid arthritis. Similarly, the 1 of our patients who had definite aortic insufficiency had an atypical picture for SLE with spondylitis consistent with rheumatoid spondylitis but without x-ray changes. Facial rash and kidney disease characteristic of SLE were present. Reported instances of aortic valvular involvement in SLE have increased in number recently [11, 29, 38, 106, 119]. In the 2 patients with aortic insufficiency seen by us since the series was closed, the disease was entirely typical.

Evidence of more frequent involvement of valves was found on postmortem examination, with some abnormality in 41% (24 of 58), an incidence more comparable with some other series [15, 16, 38, 55, 57, 93, 95, 106, 119, 131]. The mitral valve alone was involved in all but 7 cases, in which in addition the tricuspid was involved in 4, associated with the pulmonic in 1, and the aortic valve was involved in 3. In all except 2 cases the changes were similar to those first described by Libman and Sacks [153] with small verrucous vegetations chiefly on the ventricular side of the valve. They consisted usually of dense connective tissue, often some fibrinoid necrosis, slight to moderate cellular reaction usually lymphocytic, and occasional myxoid material, or slight calcification. Hematoxylin bodies were seen in 3 cases. The valvulitis in 4 cases seemed to be entirely "healed," with no evidence of active inflammation. The other two cases differed from those of Libman and Sacks, with larger vegetations spread more diffusely over the valve. Thickening of the valve or annulus or chordae tendinae was noted in 12 other patients in whom no vegetations were present. Mitral stenosis was found in 1 case. In the patient who had definite aortic insufficiency the aortic valve was thickened, up to 3 mm, with the edges rolled, and showed foci of calcification and dense fibrosis. The mitral valve and chordae tendinae also showed similar marked thickening, with foci of calcification on the mitral valve. Only occasionally was the valvulitis of sufficient degree to have produced clinical signs. Even when vegetations similar to those described by Libman and Sacks [153] were present, murmurs greater than grade 2 were heard in only 5 of the patients. This is consistent with the observation of most investigators [69, 90, 102].

Superimposed subacute bacterial endocarditis was diagnosed clinically in 2 patients, both of whom responded to treatment. Since many of the signs and symptoms of bacterial endocarditis are identical with those of the underlying lupus, diagnosis can be made only with positive blood cultures and confirmatory signs and symptoms and response to treatment. In some cases it is impossible to determine during life whether superimposed bacterial endocarditis is present. Acute bacterial endocarditis was present at postmortem in 4 cases on the valves and in 1 on the ventricular wall. The organisms were Staphylococcus aureus in 2, hemolytic streptococcus in 1, and nonhemolytic streptococcus in 2. One patient died in 1932; another died in 1940 at a time when possible antibiotic therapy was limited to sulfonamides, which were not often used in lupus patients because of the danger of a severe reaction. A third patient died in 1948 and received only 200,000 to 400,000 units of penicillin for 4 weeks.

Arrhythmia was rare, occurring in only a few patients. A low incidence has been reported by others [38, 114, 118].

Cardiac failure was not common except terminally or in patients with cor pulmonale.

Cor pulmonale. Pulmonary hypertension with resulting cor pulmonale occurred in 4 patients, presumably due to vasculitis of the pulmonary vessels, in contrast to reports from other series [38, 106] in which cor pulmonale was associated wih pulmonary fibrosis. In 1 patient who died after 17 years, the pulmonary vessels showed extensive subintimal proliferation similar to the more acute changes in a patient seen since the series was closed. In the latter case, evidence of cor pulmonale was present only 1½ years before death. Postmortem examination showed marked subintimal proliferation.

Respiratory Tract

Pleurae. Pleural involvement was very common. Fluid was found by x-ray examination in 55% (73) of 133 patients, higher in incidence than in many series [69, 102, 103, 106, 279]. Pleurisy with effusion was the presenting manifestation in 1 case, as pleurisy was in some cases in other series [69, 102, 103]. A rub was heard in 23% (33) of the 142 in the series. The high incidence of pleuritis was apparent at autopsy when 93% (54 of 58) had evidence of pleural involvement, an incidence slightly higher than that in most other series [15, 55, 145, 205, 279]. Fluid was present in 33 cases and varied in volume from less than 5 to 1500 ml. Only three effusions were hemorrhagic, two in the patient who died 10 hours after valvuloplasty, and one fluid was grossly purulent. Microscopic changes were present in 24% (14 of 58),

varying in degree from small accumulations of lymphocytes and macrophages to perivascular accumulations of fibrinoid necrosis with
infiltrate of neutrophilic polymorphonuclear and mononuclear cells,
and in severe cases to extensive infiltration of inflammatory cells and a
layer of fibrinous exudate. In 1 case hematoxylin bodies were seen.
Adhesions were found in 63% (37) of the 58 cases, varying from a few
delicate apical strands to numerous fibrous, occasionally gelatinous,
strands over both lungs. Complete adhesion was present bilaterally in
only 6 cases and unilaterally in 3.

Lungs. Parenchymatous lung involvement was common. Density,
in addition to evidence of pleural fluid, was found by x-ray in 56% (74
of 133). In the majority of cases this represented pneumonitis or small
areas of atelectasis, though in a few cases it was due to cardiac failure.
Often it was impossible to determine whether the pneumonitis, seen
frequently in association with acute exacerbations, was infectious in
nature or due to lupus. The latter was not uncommonly hemorrhagic,
as found in 31% (18 of 58) at postmortem examination. It was frequently migratory, persisting a few days in one area of the lungs and
then appearing in another area. Pulmonary fibrosis of significant degree was found in 2 patients and corroborated at postmortem examination in the 1 who died. It is impossible to be sure that it represented
a manifestation of SLE, as in the cases discussed by Eisenberg et al.
[75]. Pulmonary emboli were present in 3 patients who had had
thrombophlebitis clinically. Pneumonitis was present at postmortem
examination in 62% (36 of 58). In the majority of these pneumonitis
was apparently terminal, showing scattered areas of bronchopneumonia, usually with heavy exudate of inflammatory cells, fibrin and
often red cells, but in some there were early changes with only small
groups of alveoli containing leukocytes, erythrocytes, and fibrin.
Lobar involvement was present in only 2 patients, and chronic localized pneumonitis in only 4, associated with fibrinoid degeneration in
the alveolar septa. In the 31% (18 of 58) of the autopsies in which the
pneumonitis was hemorrhagic, the areas of hemorrhage were of various sizes, comparable to the findings of Purnell et al. [205]. Abscesses,
usually multiple, were present in 12%. Infarcts were rare, occurring in
only 4 cases. Two of these were septic infarcts. Diffuse areas of atelectasis occurred in 28% (16 of 58) but no explanation was found for the
typical plate atelectases seen frequently on x-ray. Moderate to marked
pulmonary congestion was present in 39% (23 of 58), often with associated bronchopneumonia. Active tubercles were present in 2 cases, 1

of whom had been on steroids for 4 weeks before death. Changes in the vessels of the lungs were not common. Thickening of the walls of small arteries, especially of the intima, was present in 7 patients, associated with fibrinoid necrosis in 3, hematoxylin bodies in 1, and thrombi in 3. Fibrinoid foci were found in the pulmonary artery in 1 case. In the patient who had had cor pulmonale for 17 years there was severe pulmonary artery atherosclerosis with calcification. Many small branches of the pulmonary arteries showed extensive subintimal proliferation in this case, as discussed above. Similar, more marked changes have been seen recently in a patient who died with severe, more acute pulmonary hypertension and cor pulmonale.

Larynx. Laryngitis, as indicated by persistent hoarseness, was present in 13% (18) of the 142 patients. Typical changes of cricoarytenoiditis were seen by laryngoscopy in 3 patients. In others, edema of the cords was marked, as in the case reported by Scarpelli et al. [222]. Autopsy showed foci of necrosis and polymorphonuclear infiltration of the arytenoid cartilage and muscles in 1 patient. Necrotizing, ulcerative tracheitis was found at postmortem examination in 1 patient. Ulcerative lesions of the pyriform sinus were found in 1 case.

Liver

The liver was palpable in 49% (70) of the 142 patients, a much higher percentage than that usually found in rheumatoid arthritis, 7.5% [221], or in most other series of SLE [11, 57, 69, 109, 159, 216]. Jaundice was rare, as in other series, with bilirubin greater than 2 mg per 100 ml in 7% (10 of 142). In 13% (18) it was greater than 1 mg per 100 ml. However, abnormality of one or more other liver function tests was found in 66% (57) of the 86 patients in whom the tests were performed. An additional 13% (11) had only increase in the cephalin flocculation or thymol turbidity. Prothrombin was decreased in 38% (27 of 66 patients), being below 25% in 22 patients. In 5 of these it was 13% (see discussion under *Blood,* below). The most common abnormality was in serum glutamic oxalic transaminase, but other tests often abnormal were serum alkaline phosphatase and bromsulfalein excretion. Remarkably high serum levels of glutamic oxalic transaminase (up to 420 units per ml in the series and recently over 1,000 units) were found in some patients in whom there was little or no evidence of liver involvement but no clinical evidence of other source of the large amount of the enzyme. Some of the elevation may have been associated with ingestion of aspirin, but this was not studied. In 1 of the patients with a level of 420 units, no aspirin had been given. The levels often remained high as long as the disease remained very active, even for months. Cholesterol was abnormally low, below 120 mg per 100 ml, in only 1 of the 37 patients in whom it was determined, but was elevated above 300 mg in 19% (7). Esters ranged from 51 to 70% in the 5 cases in whom the tests were performed.

Biopsies. Biopsies of the liver were performed in 3 patients. One showed moderate fatty infiltration, 1 slight lymphocytic infiltration, and 1 was negative. In all 3 cases slight abnormalities of liver function tests were present. Alkaline phosphatase was elevated to 6 or 7 Bodansky units and cephalin flocculation was 4+ in all. Bromsulfalein retention was 11% in the patient with fatty infiltration.

At postmortem examination enlargement of the liver over 1800 gm was present in 40% (23) of the 58 patients, the highest weight being 2880 gm. Moderate to marked fatty infiltration was found in 44% (26 of 58), a slightly higher incidence than found in some series [90, 102, 186]. Congestion of the portal areas of moderate or severe degree was noted in 47% (27 of 58), associated with infiltration of lymphocytes, monocytes, and neutrophils in one-third of the cases with congestion. Severe cardiac cirrhosis was present in 2 cases (1 of whom had had cor pulmonale for 17 years). An abscess, 5 cm in diameter, was present in 1 patient who had B. pyocyaneus septicemia. Hematoxylin bodies were noted in 3 cases. Hemosiderosis occurred in 1 patient who had had many transfusions over a long period of time. Only a few vessels showed thickening of the walls and perivascular infiltration of inflammatory cells. Healed arteritis was recognized in 1 case. The changes in the liver were relatively slight compared with the definite evidence of dysfunction found clinically in 66% (57) of 86 cases.

Pancreas

Clinical evidence of pancreatitis was not found in any of the patients of this series. However, amylase levels as high as 250 units per 100 ml occurred and often persisted for many months until the activity of the disease subsided.

The pancreas was not studied in detail at postmortem, but it showed very few changes, even in patients who received prednisone. The doses, however, were usually relatively low. It was normal grossly and in routine sections in all but 9 patients. In 3 there was moderate fibrosis; in 2 slight lymphocytic infiltration; in 1 diffuse ectasia of the acini; and in 3 inflammatory changes in the vessels with fibrinoid necrosis and infiltration of neutrophils and lymphocytes in the vessel walls. A small necrotic area surrounded by fibrous tissue was found in 1 patient. The absence of marked pancreatitis, in contrast to the cases discussed by Dubois [69], is of special interest since the patients in this series had received rather little steroid therapy.

Spleen

The spleen was palpable at some time in 46% (65) of the 142 patients, an incidence higher than that found in other series [69, 102, 119]. In many cases the splenomegaly persisted during periods of only slight activity of the disease, but in periods of remission the spleen was usually not palpable. Confirmation of a high incidence of splenomegaly was found at autopsy, where it was present in 67% (39) of the 58 patients. Enlargement of the spleen, either clinically or at postmortem examination, showed some correlation with hemoglobin concentration ($p = 0.017$). Only 15% (9) of the 59 patients without splenomegaly had hemoglobin levels of 8 gm/100 ml or lower, whereas 34% (27) of the 79 with enlargement of the spleen detected by clinical examination or at autopsy or by both means had levels of 8 gm or below. Of the group without splenomegaly 39% (23 of 59) had hemoglobin levels between 8 and 12 gm and 25% (20) of the 79 patients in whom enlargement was detected. There was no correlation between splenomegaly and leukocyte counts or platelet levels. The indications for splenectomy and the attendant dangers will be discussed later.

Examination of the spleen by biopsy or after removal was made in 5 patients. In general, the abnormalities were less than those found at postmortem. Three cases were entirely negative, 1 showed only basophilic material in the follicles, and the other showed fibrosis and hemosiderosis. The spleen weighed over 200 gm at postmortem in 67% (39 of 58), in addition to the 4 patients in whom splenectomy had been performed. The greatest weight was 900 gm. The most frequent abnormality was moderate to marked congestion, occurring in 33% (19 of 58), with associated infiltration of neutrophils and lymphocytes in a few cases and occasionally areas of fibrinoid necrosis or fibrosis. The arterioles showed "onion skin" thickening in 38% (22 of 58), with the width of the fibrosis equaling ⅓ the radius of the vessel. Splenic infarcts, which were always small, were found in only 10 cases. An old focus of caseation, presumably tuberculous in origin, was found in 1 patient. The Malpighian corpuscles in only a few cases showed infiltration of monocytic phagocytes and in a few patients nonspecific "toxic" changes in the center of the corpuscles. The follicles were prominent in many cases, and in many there was increased hemosiderin.

Salivary and Lacrimal Glands

Salivary and, rarely, lacrimal gland enlargement was present in 12% (17) of the 142 patients. It was occasionally associated with marked redness, tenderness, and swelling, suggesting a cellulitis. The incidence of salivary gland involvement is comparable to that of some other series [232, 233]. Sjögren's syndrome with keratoconjunctivitis sicca and/or dry mouth was relatively uncommon, occurring in only 3 of the series, comparable to the incidence reported by Dubois [69]. Eight cases of Sjögren's syndrome and SLE were reported by Steinberg and Talal [252] and one by Bain [17]. The incidence was much lower than that in series of patients with rheumatoid arthritis. It was found by Stenstam [253] in 11% of rheumatoid patients and in 9 to 34% by Bloch and Bunim [30]. Biopsy of a salivary gland in 2 patients in this series was consistent with Sjögren's syndrome. Parotid glands were enlarged in 2 patients in the series, comparable to the observations of Steinberg and Talal [252].

Vasomotor Involvement

Vasomotor abnormalities were present in 33% (32) of the 97 patients on whom information was available. The usual symptoms and signs were excessive coldness and often sweating of hands or feet. In many cases the signs appeared with the onset or exacerbation of the disease and subsided partially or entirely with remission. The total incidence is much lower than that found in patients with rheumatoid arthritis, 67% [234], but higher than that in a control series, 24% [234]. Results in SLE as reported by others vary greatly. Severe abnormalities with a picture characteristic of Raynaud's syndrome were found in 9 of the 97 patients in this series on whom adequate information was available, and less severe in 3 others, with an incidence (12%) similar to that in rheumatoid arthritis (11%) [234] but lower than that in other series of SLE [11, 69, 102, 103, 158], and higher than in controls (3%) [234]. It represented the first sign of the disease in 10 patients and persisted for 1 to 4 years before other manifestations occurred in 5 patients. In many of the severe cases, ulcerations and occasionally extensive areas of necrosis were found on fingers and occasionally toes. In 2 patients, loss of finger tips occurred spontaneously;

in 1 other amputation was performed. It has been found advisable to wait for weeks or months if necessary for spontaneous healing. The relatively good response to conservative therapy, the tendency toward poor response to sympathectomy, and the likelihood of exacerbation of lupus following sympathectomy will be discussed later, as will the possible relationship of the ulcerations to steroid therapy. Seventeen patients developed gangrenous lesions in other areas: upper arms, legs, buttocks, face and ears, and over malleoli, presumably due to localized vasculitis, though such involvement was proved by biopsy in only 1 case. Frequently, severe pain and burning accompanied these lesions, and reduction in these symptoms heralded improvement, even though objective signs had not changed. Similar cases are reviewed by Dubois [69].

Thrombophlebitis in femoral veins occurred in 7 of the patients in this series. In 3 of them pulmonary emboli were found at postmortem examination. The incidence of thrombophlebitis was much lower than that found by Alarcón-Segovia and Osmundsom [7].

Vasculitis

It is apparent that widespread vasculitis, which has been demonstrated in many cases of this series and others by biopsy or autopsy, explains many of the symptoms and signs of SLE. Outstanding are the palmar and finger-tip lesions, the skin ulcers, mouth ulcers, many lesions of the central and peripheral nervous system, and the malignant hypertension in some patients. Vasculitis caused beginning gangrene of the distal 2 feet of the ileum in one patient, comparable to reports in the literature [27, 39, 200]. Vasculitis in vessels other than the glomerular capillaries and splenic arterioles, discussed above, occurred in 51% (30) of the 58 patients. Commonly, in 18% (10), the vessels of many organs were involved, as reported by others [15, 55, 57, 131], but in other cases the inflammatory vascular changes were limited to one or a few organs, including kidneys, testis, ovaries, brain and spinal cord, pulmonary artery, portal vessels, lymph nodes, serosa, liver, gallbladder, stomach, synovial tissue, skin, vasa vasorum of the aorta, and the aorta itself. The involvement varied from small foci in cross sections of the vessel to complete involvement, and from changes in the intima or adventitia only to abnormalities of all three layers. Histologic findings were usually thickening of the intima and media, often with infiltration of neutrophils, lymphocytes, and plasma cells and with areas of fibrinoid necrosis, and perivascular infiltration of monocytes, lymphocytes, and plasma cells. In a few cases capillaries showed endothelial proliferation. A loose lamellar fibrous reaction in the adventitia was noted in 1 case, and "onion skin" thickening in the adventitia of stomach vessels in another. In 6 severe cases with necrotizing arteritis the changes were indistinguishable from those found in periarteritis nodosa, as was well indicated in 1 of these cases discussed by Weiss and Mallory in 1938 [276]. Inflammatory changes were found in coronary vessels in 3 patients, 2 of whom had had myocardial infarctions. The changes varied from moderate intimal proliferation and infiltration of plasma cells, monocytes, and lymphocytes in the media and adventitia, to severe necrotizing arteritis. In the patient who had had a myocardial infarction at the age of 27, 1 year before death, there was acute inflammation and necrosis of the intima and media near the old thrombus area and in one area of the right coronary. Femoral or popliteal veins showed thrombophlebitis in 3 cases. Two had had pulmonary emboli and one had also a thrombus in the left pulmonary artery. One of these 2 had had ligation of the superficial femoral veins. Acute and chronic phlebitis with an organizing thrombus was present in the jugular vein in 1 case.

Atherosclerosis was found in 6 patients, generalized in 2, and localized to the aorta in 2 and to the aorta and renal arteries in another. Severe atherosclerosis of the pulmonary arteries was present in the patient who had had cor pulmonale for 17 years. It is of interest that the small branches showed extensive subintimal proliferation.

Chemical and Immunological Features

Blood

Leukocytes. One of the most characteristic laboratory findings was leukopenia. A white cell count of 4,000 per cu mm or less was present on at least two occasions in 67% (95 of 142), the lowest being 450 with an absolute neutrophil count of 300. This incidence is similar to that reported in most series. In only 12% (17) was the count always between 4,000 and 10,000. In 22% (31) it was above 10,000 at some time and in 16% (23) it was above 20,000 at some time. A leukocyte count above 30,000 was rare, however, occurring in only 4 patients, usually terminally. The highest count in the series was 99,500 in a patient with pneumococcal lobar pneumonia. The presence of leukopenia adds weight to a diagnosis of lupus, whereas high counts above 30,000, such as those occasionally seen in rheumatoid arthritis, make the diagnosis of lupus very unlikely.

The percentage of neutrophils usually remains relatively normal, being less than 50% in only 26% (37) of the 142 in this series. However, in many cases an increase to 90% was found at times as in other series [69, 179]. The absolute number of neutrophils is therefore presumably adequate even with total leukocyte counts of 2,000 or less. This conclusion is consistent with the fact that patients with lupus not treated with steroids or cytotoxic drugs probably have only a somewhat greater susceptibility to infection, though they do tend to have exacerbations with infections [191]. In a study under very limited conditions Staples et al. [248] found an increased number of infections in lupus patients not treated with steroids.

Eosinophils. Abnormal percentages of eosinophils (greater than 5%) were found at some time in 21% (30) of the 142 patients, a slightly higher incidence that that in other series [102, 103, 239]. The highest percentage was 48% with a leukocyte count of 11,500 per cu mm persisting for many days during a severe exacerbation.

Platelets. Platelets were reduced in number in 17% (24) of the series of 142, the lowest count being 2,500, and counts as low as 7,000 have been seen rarely in other patients. Actual counts were made in 18% (25) of the series, a reduction in the number of platelets being estimated in the other patients by examination of several blood smears. The incidence is slightly higher than in some series [69, 102, 103, 146], although reports vary. The greatest reductions in this series were usually found in acute exacerbation with "crisis," though occasionally the thrombocytopenia, with very low levels of platelets and associated purpura, was the first manifestation of the disease. Often in such cases few or no other signs of the disease appeared immediately. Of the 23 patients with reduced number of platelets, 15 had purpura. The effect of splenectomy and other treatments will be discussed later.

In this series there is no information as to the "adhesiveness" of the platelets in each patient and the subsequent effect on bleeding. In a few cases bleeding occurred at reduced but rather unexpectedly high levels of platelets. In such cases it seems possible that the platelet aggregation was lessened, though measurements were not made. Various drugs have been demonstrated to reduce platelet aggregation, one of which is aspirin [257], commonly used in the treatment of systemic lupus. In contrast, platelet counts as low as 2,500 were present in one patient with no evidence of bleeding. In some patients in whom bleeding occurred with relatively high platelet counts the bleeding was apparently related to a circulating anticoagulant. Tests for circulating anticoagulants were carried out in only a few of the patients of this series. As found by others [35, 69, 167, 286], more than one anticoagulant may be present. In one patient, anti-factor X was found. In another patient seen since the series ended, two circulating anticoagulants were found. One was the relatively typical one against prothrombin activator, the other a separate antithrombin which is present in about one-third of the patients who have the above anticoagulant. A lowering of prothrombin or partial thromboplastin time [46] should make one suspicious of a circulating anticoagulant and requires a search for one.

Hemoglobin. A marked reduction in hemoglobin is also a common manifestation of lupus. In this series, 8% (11 of 142) had less than 6 gm per 100 ml at some time, the lowest being 3.4 gm, and another 18% (26) less than 8 gm. However, 49% (70 of 142) had levels over 12 gm at all times, a higher incidence than in most series [69, 102, 179]. Since levels below 8 gm are unusual in patients with rheumatoid arthritis, a low value is often helpful in suggesting lupus when the differential lies between these two diseases. In the majority of patients with lupus, the lowering in the hemoglobin level is due to hemolysis.

Hemolysis (as defined as a reticulocyte count greater than 1%, a urobilinogen greater than 1 Ehrlich unit or a drop of 6 in the hematocrit in a few days) occurred in 67% (46) of the 68 patients on whom information was available. In all but 8 patients (6%) the reticulocyte count was above 2% or the urobilinogen above 2. The incidence of hemolysis is much higher than that of 16% (39 of 245) found in the study of patients for the determination of the criteria for classification of SLE [51]. In the same study the incidence in RA was 2.6%. During acute exacerbations or crises, the drop in hematocrit may be very rapid (over 5% in a few days) without obvious blood loss. Confirmatory evidence of hemolysis was present in the reticulocyte counts of 9 and 12% in 2 of the 3 patients in our series with sudden drops in hematocrit. The incidence of severe hemolytic anemia was comparable to that in other series [69, 179]. The highest reticulocyte count in our series was 44% and the highest urobilinogen was 38 Ehrlich units. More commonly, during moderately active disease, a low degree of hemolysis is present with reticulocyte counts a little above normal (2% to 8%) and often normal urobilinogen. In such cases the hematocrit remains at a constant level (for example, 25%). If raised by transfusions (to 30 or 32%), it will again remain constant and not fall to the previous level, suggesting a constant rate of production just equal to that of hemolysis but not adequate to raise the hemoglobin in the presence of the hemolysis. Haptoglobins were looked for in only a few patients. The level was reduced in the presence of hemolysis, as would be expected. Folic acid deficiency was noted in only 2 patients but few were examined.

In occasional cases iron lack is, at least in part, the etiological factor in the anemia in lupus and must always be sought when hemoglobin rise is slow.

Coombs test, performed in only 58 patients, was positive in 28% (16). Hemolysis occurred in 81% (13) of the 16 patients with positive Coombs test, but also in 60% (25) of the 42 patients with negative Coombs tests.

Sedimentation Rate

The erythrocyte sedimentation rate was elevated in the patients with active disease. It ranged from 0.13 mm per min to 2.2 mm by a method in which the upper limit of normal is 0.35 mm per min [217]. The rate correlated with the activity of the disease in most cases and decreased markedly or returned to normal remission, as was reported by Armas-Cruz et al. [11].

Serum Proteins

Serum globulin concentration as determined by ammonium sulfate precipitation was elevated in 73% (77) of the 106 patients in whom it was determined. In 44% (47) it was between 3.0 and 4.0 gm/100 ml, and in 29% (31) greater than 4.0 gm. In only 5 patients, however, was the concentration greater than 5 gm/100 ml. The duration of disease in these patients was 22 years or more. The incidence of elevated levels was higher than in most other series.

Marked lowering of the albumin concentration occurred in many patients, usually associated with significant proteinuria and with edema. In a few cases, serum concentrations as low as 2.0 gm per 100 ml were found in patients who had had no detected loss of albumin in the urine. Whether or not this was due to liver dysfunction, as seems possible, was not apparent. In one such patient, SGOT was 25 units per 100 ml, bromsulfalein retention was 9%, and cephalin flocculation was negative in 48 hours.

Electrophoretic pattern of proteins. Electrophoretic pattern of proteins was abnormal in 73% (52) of the 73 patients in whom it was determined. Twenty-nine percent (21) had elevated γ-globulin concentrations and 19% (14) had elevated a2 globulins. The highest levels were 37% of γ globulin, equivalent to a concentration of 2.6 gm per 100 ml, and 13% of a2 globulins, equivalent to 1 gm per 100 ml. The incidence of abnormalities was lower than in most series.

Immunoglobulins. Immunoglobulins were not examined during this study. In other studies elevation of IγG has predominated, though increase in IγM and IγA has been present, also, in a large proportion of patients with SLE [45, 87]. A marked acceleration in the turnover of IγG in SLE was shown by Levy et al. [150].

Serological tests for syphilis. Hinton or Wasserman tests were positive in 18% (19) of the 106 patients in whom they were performed. Treponema pallidum inhibition tests were not known during the first half of this study. The results have been negative in the patients with positive serological tests in whom the TPI test has been done. In none of the other patients was there any suggestion of syphilis by history or examination. The incidence of false positive tests for syphilis has been reported in varied percentages but often in the same percentage as in this series [57, 60, 137, 216]. The fact that the positive test may precede clinical evidence of systemic lupus by many years was indicated by the studies of Moore and Lutz [185]. None of our patients have had fluorescent treponema antibody absorption tests, which were found by Kraus et al. [138] to be "beaded with SLE and not with syphilis."

LE cells. LE cells were found on at least two occasions in 58% (51) of the 87 patients on whom the test was performed. In another 29% (25) LE cells were seen on one occasion. However, in 13% (11) no definite or suspicious LE cells were seen at any time. The criteria for acceptance of an LE cell as "definite" were strict. The phagocytosed material had to be entirely homogeneous, with no suggestion of residual discrete chromatin. Suspicious cells might have slight variations in staining of the material, but still no suggestion of an intact nucleus such as that seen in nuclear phagocytosis.

The incidence of LE cells in this series may have been reduced slightly by the fact that in some of the patients on whom the tests were performed, soon after the first description of LE cells by Hargraves et al. [101], the disease had already gone into remission. In others seen at that time only a few tests could be performed during the follow-up and the technique of the test was not well known to us then. However, a somewhat comparable incidence has been found by most of the

investigators who do not use a positive LE cell test as an essential cri-
terion for the diagnosis of SLE [11, 57, 69, 220, 233].

A finding of LE cells in the blood does not make a diagnosis of lupus
since they occur in 4 to 27% of patients with rheumatoid arthritis [11,
81, 100, 108, 148, 268], in other generalized connective tissue diseases
[156], in other diseases such as hepatitis and ulcerative colitis [5], and
may be produced by many medications, including hydralazine, procainamide, diphenylhydantoin, and tridione [33, 71, 73, 197, 285].
Therefore many investigators do not require a positive LE cell test for
a diagnosis of SLE, evaluating it as only one of several criteria which
in combination make a diagnosis of lupus as definite as is possible in
the absence of any proof of the disease. There is surely no evidence
that treatment should be changed in any way because of the finding of
an LE cell.

The presence of LE cells correlated with the number of joints involved ($p = 0.02$). Eighty-four percent (64) of the 76 patients with
positive LE cell tests had more than 3 joints involved, in contrast to
44% (5) of the 11 with negative tests. Twelve percent (9) of those with
LE cells had less than 3 joints involved but 44% (5) of those in whom
no LE cells were seen. There was a correlation also with the presence
of casts ($p = 0.007$). Sixty-seven percent (7) of the patients with negative LE tests had no casts but only 19% of the 76 with LE cells. Forty-
one percent (31) of the latter had more than occasional casts, in contrast to 22% (2) of the 11 patients without LE cells. No correlation was
found with age of onset, pain in joints, albuminuria without infection,
hematuria, hemoglobin concentration, globulin levels, latex test for
rheumatoid factor, course, severity, duration of disease, or number of
patients who died.

The percentage of positive tests for LE cells that return to normal
when the disease goes into remission could not be determined in this
series since the tests were not repeated regularly in the majority of
cases. However, in 11 patients LE cells disappeared with remission. In
2 cases the test first became positive with an exacerbation of the disease. A disappearance of positive tests with remissions has been found
in some cases by others [104, 215].

Antinuclear antibodies. The majority of the patients in this series
were seen before the determination of antinuclear antibodies (ANA)
was available. Therefore no information can be obtained from them
as to the incidence of positive ANA in SLE or as to its relationship to
course, characteristics, or prognosis. However, evidence from our

subsequent experience and reports from many investigators indicate that antinuclear antibodies are almost universally present in patients with SLE. It is important to realize, however, that their absence does not rule out the diagnosis of SLE if it is adequately supported by other criteria, as will be discussed in Chapter 3 under Differential Diagnosis. Antinuclear antibodies are relatively nonspecific and found in many conditions [19]. Incidence in rheumatoid arthritis is high [20], for instance.

In few of this series have determinations of anti-DNA antibodies or of free DNA been made, so no statements can be made as to the incidence or relationship to course or characteristics. However, observations since those first recorded in 1957 have indicated a high incidence of antibodies to DNA in SLE [112, 226], and of DNA at periods in the disease [113].

Nuclear fluorescence. The immunofluorescent patterns vary in their association with different diseases but any one may occur in SLE and no one is specific, in contrast to the findings of Gonzalez and Rothfield [87]. The patterns are summarized as follows by Bloch and Helms [31]. The homogeneous pattern may be attributed to antibody directed against particulate nucleoprotein and is frequently seen in SLE. The nuclear rim pattern may be attributed to antibody to DNA and to antibody to soluble nucleoprotein. The presence of either antibody shows a high correlation with active SLE, particularly with active lupus nephritis. The speckled pattern may be attributed to antibody directed against a saline-soluble component of the nucleus devoid of nucleic acids or histones. This is probably the least specific, being seen with sera from many diseases including SLE. The nucleolar pattern may be attributed to antibody directed against nucleolar RNA. Initially reported in high incidence in serum of patients with scleroderma, this antibody has also been identified in SLE.

Rheumatoid factor. Rheumatoid factor was present in 50% (71) of the 142 patients. The highest titer was 1:5,120 by latex fixation. The incidence in other series varies from 15 to 80%, partly according to the method used [60, 69, 109]. There was no correlation with renal involvement, as indicated by casts or red cells in the urine, or with positive tests for LE cells.

Complement components. Complement components, either CH_{50} or C_3, were determined in only a small number of the patients of this series so that no conclusions can be drawn from them. However, in several cases increase or decrease in the complement levels correlated well with changes in activity of the disease. As found by other investigators [199, 225, 226], the correlation was better with renal or skin disease than with other signs of activity. However, changes in complement levels in some cases reflected also alterations in activity of disease as manifested in other systems. In 1 patient, for instance, the occurrence of psychosis following a period of remission without other clinical evidence of disease activity was reflected in a 35% lowering of the level of CH_{50} as well as increase in sedimentation rate and decrease in hemoglobin level. B_1A (B_1C) globulin levels were found by Miyasato et al. [181] to be lower in patients with active disease. Other investigators [98, 199] found lower spinal fluid C_4 in patients with central nervous system involvement. Total complement was reduced in synovial fluids in SLE studied by Pekin and Zvaifler [198]. The serum complement level did not always reflect the activity of the disease and a decrease in complement should not be used alone as an indication for treatment with steroids or cytotoxic drugs.

The lowered complement level in SLE is assumed to arise from the fixation of complement by immune complexes. Uninterpretable are the very high levels seen in occasional patients with rapid progression of disease to death in several months but with no evidence of infection. In our experience this has occurred notably in 2 patients with excessively high blood pressure levels and little evidence of glomerulitis. At postmortem examination, in 1 case, the glomeruli showed minimal proliferative changes, but other vessels showed moderately severe inflammation.

Body Fluids

Synovial fluid. Synovial fluid examinations were performed in 11 patients. The most striking finding was the relatively slight indication of inflammation. Leukocyte counts were extremely low, ranging from 100 to 3,000 with an average of 1,060 per cu mm in the absence of infection. The absolute count of neutrophilic polymorphonuclears was almost always below 1,000 as in several other series [110, 198, 247]. In a few cases seen since the series ended, the total white count was 10,000 per cu mm, but the percentage of polymorphonuclears was very low. Only with infection were significantly elevated leukocyte counts found. The low absolute count of neutrophils is so characteristic that one should be extremely hesitant to make a diagnosis of SLE when the count is high in the absence of infection (as for instance 10,000 with 50% polymorphonuclears). Similarly, mucin precipitates were always normal with tight clumps and clear surrounding solution, and relative viscosity was correspondingly high, usually above normal, in great contrast to the usual findings in rheumatoid arthritis [210] but comparable to those in other series of SLE [34, 198, 247]. Sugar concentration was essentially the same as that in the serum. Total protein levels were only slightly above normal. LE cells were not looked for in all fluids but in an occasional fluid that had stood at room temperature before examination typical LE cells were found.

Pericardial, pleural, and peritoneal fluids. The surprisingly low absolute number of neutrophils in synovial fluid is duplicated in pericardial, pleural, and peritoneal fluid in SLE. Usually the number is much less than 1,000 cells per cu mm in any fluid unless there is superimposed infection. The average leukocyte counts were 1,600, 590, and 100 per cu mm in 3 pericardial, 6 pleural, and 2 peritoneal fluids. In a pericardial and pleural fluid in 1 patient at postmortem, high counts (30,000 and 14,000 per cu mm) were found following tamponade, aspiration, and bleeding. In 1 other patient pericardial and pleural fluid counts were high, 31,000 and 11,500 with 92% and 72% neutrophils. Infection was not proved but was suspected. LE cells were seen in 1 pericardial fluid. A low leukocyte count (300 per cu mm) with no neutrophils was found in ascitic fluid by Friedberg et al. [79].

Cerebrospinal fluids. Cerebrospinal fluids were examined in 35 patients. Twenty-one were normal with usually 2 cells and always less than 8 cells, mostly lymphocytes, and with protein concentrations of less than 50 mg per 100 ml. In 4 of these cases colloidal gold results were 0122210000. In 2 others colloidal gold tests were 2221000000 and 1222454211 with otherwise normal findings. In 1 fluid obtained after a seizure the colloidal gold was 5552200000. Leukocyte counts were elevated to 26 and 100 cells per cu mm in 2 other patients, and in another, who developed peripheral neuritis following tetanus antitoxin, the cell count was 5,700 per cu mm. In 8 other patients, protein levels were elevated, varying from 53 to 240 mg per 100 ml. The level of complement (C_4) has been found to be low in other series [98, 199].

Hematoxylin Bodies

Hematoxylin bodies were noted in 14% (8) of the 58 cases at postmortem, being found most commonly in kidney and liver, but also in spleen, lymph nodes, pleura, mitral valve (3), pericardial vessels, endocardium, jugular vein, small vessels in the alveolar walls, lungs, muscle, synovial tissues, and bone marrow. They were found by Gross [93] chiefly in the heart, especially the valves.

3 Diagnosis

Unless the typical butterfly rash or a combination of characteristic manifestations as listed in Chapter 1 under the criteria for this series is present, diagnosis is often difficult and many diseases must be included in the differential. In patients with gradual onset of disease and, at first, largely systemic manifestations such as malaise, fatiguability, weakness, slight fever, and slight intermittent aching, the possibility of diseases such as tuberculosis or other chronic infections, lymphoma or other generalized malignancies, thyrotoxicosis, psychogenic disorders, and any of the so-called generalized connective tissue diseases must be considered. However, the course in most patients, with appearance of a more characteristic picture and the persistent absence of corroborating evidence for the other diagnoses, leads to a definite diagnosis usually within weeks or months. The finding of LE cells in the blood at this stage adds only further suggestion of the disease and does not make possible a diagnosis of SLE until further characteristic findings appear.

Differential Diagnosis

In general, the diseases from which it is most difficult to differentiate SLE are rheumatoid arthritis and the vasculitides. Only rarely is there persistent difficulty in separating rheumatic fever or dermatomyositis from SLE. Scleroderma offers no difficulty except in the early stages. But differentiation from rheumatoid arthritis (RA) may not be possible for months or years and in a few cases can not be made. The resemblance of a patient with rheumatoid arthritis, manifested by severe malaise, fever, polyarthritis, pericarditis, pleurisy, and perhaps even LE cells, to a patient with SLE is great and is often confusing.

This picture probably represents one of the reasons why patients are wrongly included in reported series of SLE.

Most helpful in differentiation from rheumatoid arthritis is the presence of a typical lupus rash in butterfly distribution or a glomerulonephritis. In the case of the rash, psoriasis and acne must be ruled out, and in relation to the renal involvement the possibility exists of an acute poststreptococcal glomerulonephritis occurring concurrently with rheumatoid arthritis. However, the presence of a typical rash or nephritis adds great weight to the diagnosis of SLE, and when both are present most of the criteria are satisfied. Another finding that supports the diagnosis of SLE is a hemoglobin of less than 8 gm per 100 ml (found in only a small percent in rheumatoid arthritis). Hemolytic anemia does occur in rheumatoid arthritis but in a small percentage of patients as compared to that in SLE, 67% (46 of 68) in this series. Thrombocytopenia also supports the diagnosis of SLE since it is extremely rare in RA if it even occurs, and is relatively common in SLE, 17% (24 of 142) in this series. A leukocyte count below 4,000 per cu mm adds weight to the diagnosis of SLE, though patients with RA often have leukopenia and may occasionally have a white count as low as 1,000 per cu mm. A count above 30,000 is extremely rare in SLE, found at any time in only 4 patients in this series, but may occur more frequently in RA, especially in children. Elevated total leukocyte and neutrophilic polymorphonuclear cell counts in joint fluid (above 5,000 or 1,000 cells per cu mm respectively) tend to rule out SLE unless there is infection in the joint. Similarly, elevated polymorphonuclear cell counts in pleural or pericardial fluid are rarely found in SLE in the absence of infection, but occur usually in RA. Fever is, in general, more marked in SLE than in RA, except in children. Hair loss found in 46% (63 of 138) in this series is relatively rare in RA (4%) [51]. Sensitivity to sun is much more common in SLE, 34% (48 of 142) in this series, than in RA (1%) [51].

The presence of LE cells in the blood does not make the diagnosis of SLE. It represents one other corroborating finding, but adequate other criteria must be present. LE cells have been reported in 4 to 27% of patients with RA [11, 81, 100, 108, 148, 268]. As discussed above, LE cells are found, also, in patients with hepatitis, dermatomyositis, and in sensitivity to drugs such as penicillin, and after treatment with hydralazine, procainamide, diphenylhydantoin and tridione in some cases. Rheumatoid factor is of little value in the differential diagnosis of SLE and RA in any individual patient. Positive tests by bentonite or latex fixations occur much more commonly in RA but are found in many patients with SLE, as in 50% (71 of 142) in this series. Similarly, antinuclear antibodies are of little value in any one patient since they occur so commonly in RA. However, a negative test makes SLE unlikely.

Differentiation of SLE from the vasculitides is sometimes difficult because there is such generalized vasculitis in SLE, with resulting similarity of manifestations. However, the presence of typical rash, hemolytic anemia, thrombocytopenia, hair loss, sun sensitivity and serositis leads to the diagnosis of SLE, whereas development of one of the characteristic syndromes of vasculitis rules out SLE.

Relationship of Discoid to Systemic Lupus

The relationship of discoid to systemic lupus erythematosus has been a subject of controversy for years. Kaposi [126] in 1872 stated that chronic discoid lupus may exacerbate with acute eruption and occasionally death. However, thirty years ago the opinion that they were separate diseases was expressed by a majority of authors. In recent years there has been an increasingly large, and now probably predominant, number of investigators who consider discoid lupus to be one stage or type of SLE.

Outstanding in the arguments against the theory that the two are the same disease is the evidence that the skin lesions in discoid lupus are less florid, slow in progression, usually discrete, and productive of much atrophy and scarring. The absence of significant systemic involvement is often considered further indication that discoid and systemic lupus are separate. However, in contrast, some investigators have noted the many, relatively minor, signs of systemic disease (such as elevated sedimentation rate, fever, arthralgias, paresthesias, leukopenia, and often the presence of LE cells) in patients with discoid lupus [25, 142, 228], and in some cases have argued that this explains the apparent overlap between two separate diseases.

Strong evidence for the unity of the two is the frequency with which patients with discoid lupus develop typical SLE. In 16% (23) of the 142 of the present series discoid lesions appeared first and the characteristic systemic disease developed after periods varying from a few weeks to 22 years. Similar findings have been reported from many series [69,

97, 129, 183, 206, 213, 228, 233, 271]. Lesions entirely characteristic of discoid lupus occasionally develop at any time during the course of SLE. The similarity of lesions from patients diagnosed as "discoid lupus" and those with SLE has been noted by pathologists. In one of our histologic reports, comment was made on the fact that the lesions differ only in chronicity and fibrosis. A similar opinion has been expressed by others [*25, 69, 206, 213*], who have reported that biopsies of lesions in patients with systemic lupus were like those of discoid.

The present knowledge of discoid and systemic lupus would be well explained by the theory that they are stages of one disease. The "discoid" stage represents disease of relatively low activity, with slow progression and with chronic skin lesions. Fully developed SLE is usually a disease of greater activity and widespread systemic involvement, with more acute inflammatory changes in the skin in most cases. All stages of overlap are seen, ranging from patients with clear-cut discoid lesions and minimal systemic involvement to those with typical systemic lupus erythematosus and small areas of discoid lesions.

The prognosis in patients whose disease starts as "discoid lupus" is probably better than in those with onset as widespread disease. However, there is no proof of this. In our series, 16% (23) started as discoid lupus and only 2 had died at the end of the study, with durations of disease from onset ranging from 6½ to 54 years.

Associated Diseases

A great variety of other diseases occurred during the course of SLE in these 142 patients. In some cases, the associated disease probably resulted from the pathogenetic mechanisms of SLE itself, as with thyroiditis and Sjögren's disease. In some, no interrelationship is apparent. Other conditions were presumably related to or enhanced by therapy, as for example, bleeding peptic ulcers, or tuberculosis in 1 patient. Infections of many types were associated, as discussed above.

Active focal pulmonary tuberculosis was found at autopsy in 2 patients, one of whom was receiving steroids. One other patient had had tuberculosis of one knee and of the peritoneum at the age of 3 to 4, 9 years before the onset of SLE.

Thyroiditis was shown by biopsy in 3 patients and at postmortem examination in 3 cases. Significant enlargement of the thyroid was present in 16 patients. Thyroid activity in these patients varied from definite myxedema to hyperthyroidism but the majority were euthyroid.

Sjögren's disease was present in only 3 patients and the findings on biopsy in 2 of these cases were typical. However, enlargement of the salivary glands was found in 14 others. A similarly low incidence of Sjögren's disease, in contrast to the relatively high percentage found in rheumatoid arthritis [30, 253], has been reported by others [17, 69].

Pernicious anemia occurred in 2 patients. Thalassemia minor was present in 1 case.

Myasthenia gravis was present in 2 cases. In both, it was responsive to neostigmine. Other investigators have reported association with SLE [164, 280].

Diabetes was noted in only 1 patient.

Sarcoidosis in a skin lesion on the cheek was present in 1 patient.

Malignancies were rare in this series. One patient had a carcinoma of the breast with involvement of 19 nodes. Fifteen years later carcinoma was found in the remaining breast, perhaps from the original tumor, and widespread metastases occurred. This was not accompanied by any exacerbation of SLE. One other patient had a squamous cell carcinoma of the cheek, a third patient malignancy of the uterus, and a fourth Hodgkin's lymphoma. In 1 patient, seen since the series was closed, an oat-cell carcinoma of the lung was found. The first 4 patients received only aspirin without any steroids or cytotoxic drugs. It is of interest that 3 of them had had SLE for approximately 20 years before the malignancy developed. The medications given to the fifth patient are not known.

4 Course of the Disease

General

Long-term observation of patients with SLE reveals a seemingly infinite variety of courses. As a result, there is as yet no means of foreseeing the course either in patients in whom the activity is mild at first or in those who start with severe disease. The disease may remain mild for many years and never manifest itself in severe activity (Appendix, cases 5 and 6). Seventeen percent (24) of our series of 142 never had greater activity than the arbitrary grade of 3, and 41% (58) had grade 2 or less for the first 2 years or more. Indeed, in 9% (13) the activity never exceeded grade 2 at any time. Of the latter group 85% (11) were patients first seen after 1949. The longest duration of disease from onset in this group with mild disease was 25 years. In our series without any episode of grade 3+ activity but >2+, the longest duration of disease was 42 years and 43% lived over 15 years. Including the period of time since the series was closed, 27% have lived over 25 years.

At the other extreme from the disease of mild activity is that with severe manifestations (grade 3 to 4) very soon after onset, and a course steadily downhill or with only short remissions, and death usually within 2 to 3 years (see Appendix, cases 7 and 8). The only group of patients in whom the course is similar in all is this severe group with steadily downhill course—varying only in the rate of worsening and the presence or absence of short remissions (see Appendix, cases 9 and 10). This is the type that was seen most commonly until 20 or 25 years ago, partly because infections, which may greatly enhance the severity of an attack of lupus, were then largely uncontrollable, and probably partly because the milder stages of activity were less well recognized and diagnosis was not made until the disease became severe. However, the fact that 82% (49) of the earlier group of

60 had acute onset makes the latter explanation less likely. Of significance, also, may possibly have been the extremely pessimistic attitude of physicians regarding the outcome of the disease, often transmitted to some degree to the patients, and the resulting failure to maintain the full conservative regime even during acute exacerbations. Indicative of such reaction is the following, taken from one of our records in early 1950 of a 14-year-old girl: The family was told that the disease "is invariably fatal—that she will die from it at some date in the future, which may be a few weeks or a few months from now, and there is nothing anyone can do at present to 'cure' this disease. . . . They were advised not to bring her back to the hospital." These statements were written 27 days before the patient died. The physicians were disturbed, even though the patient was slightly better clinically, because the NPN of 88 mg/100 ml had not decreased on a relatively low dose of cortisone (400 mg for 1 day, 200 mg for 1 day and 50-100 mg for 15 days). With our present experience we know that the BUN may fall only slowly over several weeks, even though the exacerbation of the disease may be subsiding steadily with the basic regime and whatever anti-inflammatory agent is being used—occasionally with aspirin, often with corticosteroids or immunosuppressive drugs (see Chapter 5).

Review of the difference in treatment in the cases seen in the first 10 years of this study and those in the last 10 years reveals that in the earlier years there was much less emphasis on rest, and on all possible avoidance of emotional stress, as well as much less regular use of aspirin in full doses. The use of sulfonamides, with subsequent severe and occasionally fatal reactions, which was a detrimental factor in some of the earlier group, is now rarely encountered because of less widespread use of sulfonamides, and also because of the more general realization of the dangers of these drugs in SLE. Finally, it is also intriguing to speculate that the severity of the disease may have changed for reasons not yet known, as did that of other diseases such as diphtheria and rheumatic fever without any apparent changes in treatment. Of major importance in the decrease in severity is the availability of antibiotics and corticosteroids.

The severe, steadily downhill type of course was seen in 46% (28) of the 60 patients in our series who were first seen before 1949, and in only 19% (16) of the 82 first seen in 1949 or later. In addition, 60% (17) of those with the steadily downhill course first seen before 1949 died in 1 year or less with only 8% (2) living over 2 years, whereas in the later group only 19% (3) died in 1 year or less and 44% (7) lived over 2 years. As indicated above, all of the factors playing a role in the decrease in severe disease are not known. That it is not solely an effect of corticosteroid therapy is shown by the fact that only 72% (59) of the 82 patients first seen in 1949 or since received any steroids. Of the group with the severe type of course seen since steroids were available, 75% (12 of 16) received steroid therapy for periods ranging from 5 weeks to 1⅔ years. The doses varied from 40 to 100 mg of prednisone at the onset of treatment, with the exception of 2 patients in whom the initial doses were only 10 and 30 mg. The maintenance doses throughout the periods of treatment ranged from 20 to 60 mg. In the other 25% (4), the patients received steroid therapy for only 4 to 10 days before death, in doses ranging from 20 to 100 mg of prednisone.

Between the patients with relatively mild courses and those with severe downhill courses are a large number (46%) (65 of 142) in whom a great variety of courses is seen. The reasons for the variations are not clear and a prophecy as to the likely course in any one patient cannot be made. There are indications of many factors that tend to produce exacerbations, and some suggestion of those that lead to remission (as will be discussed later). The disease may start with very severe disease, grade 3 or 4, subside slowly or fairly rapidly, and remain subsequently in a stage of slight activity or remission for many years. Five percent (3) of the 60 patients first seen before 1949 and 10% (8) of the later group of 82 patients showed this course. This can happen with or without steroid therapy in the severe attack (see Appendix, cases 11 and 12). Again, in contrast, the activity may be mild (with or without exacerbations and remissions) for years (usually 3 to 5 but up to 18 years in 1 patient in our series). Then, often suddenly, it becomes severe, sometimes resulting in death. This type of course was seen in 30% (18 of 60) before 1949 and 18% (15 of 82) since (see Appendix, cases 13 and 14). A severe type of course not commonly seen is one of recurrent exacerbations for years, usually less than grade 3+ activity but occasionally 4, and relatively short remissions, usually not below grade 1 (see cases 3 and 4). This course was seen in 1 of the patients seen before 1949 and in 4 since. Of these, 4 patients died in 3 to 10 years after onset of the disease. The other patient was alive after 10 years and had been in fairly good remission for 6 years with moderate reduction of renal function. Still another course is that with several years of mild disease, then severe exacerbation for months or years, followed by another period of relatively mild disease for years (see Appendix, cases 15 and 16).

Remissions

The tendency of the disease is to remit. Even in the patients with very severe disease and, in general, a steadily downhill course, slight or moderate remissions occurred in many cases. In this series 60% of the 100 episodes called remissions, with subsidence to grade 1, were over 6 months in duration, and only 7% were less than 3 months. It seems very unwise and of no value to consider improvement for less than 2 months or at least 6 weeks as a remission, as is done by some investigators. Thirty-seven of the remissions in this series were between 3 and 10 years and 4 more were over 10 years (cases 1, 2, 11, and 12). In the 60 patients first seen before 1949, 56% (34) had remissions of some degree and in the 82 seen in 1949 or thereafter, 81% (66) had remissions. This incidence is higher than that of other investigators, even in series in which improvement for a few weeks was considered to be a remission. In 27 cases the remissions were excellent and the patients could lead relatively normal lives. In 10 of them the patients had no residual clinical or laboratory evidence of disease during the remission, other than occasionally elevated sedimentation rate and, in a few, the presence of LE cell factor or other antinuclear antibodies. These factors persisted in the majority of the few patients who were tested during remission, as has been found by others. Albuminuria in 4 cases decreased from 3 or 4+ to 0, as found, also, by Rothfield et al. [214]. Such complete remissions may last for years—up to 18 years in this series—with a slight transient exacerbation to grade 1 activity in a few patients during the period of the remission. If one includes the years since the series was closed, the longest duration of such excellent remission is 25 years. In 15 other patients the remissions were very good, with residual activity of grade 1 or less, and the patients were able to lead fairly normal lives. The longest period of remission in this group was 18 years, in a patient who has continued to be almost well in the subsequent 7 years. In 2 other patients, the clinical remissions were very good for 8 and 12 years but, in 1 case, cor pulmonale persisted and, in the other, some renal failure with an NPN of 35-45 mg/100 ml. The former patient continued to lead a fairly active life for 6 more years before death but the latter died 6 months after the long remission ended.

The amazing occurrence of excellent remissions, often lasting for years, even after severe exacerbations and actual "crisis," is well documented in this series but not yet generally known. Eleven patients lived many years (from 4 to 18 years) after such a severe flare of the disease that they were either extremely ill, grade 3 to 4, or moribund. Eight of these were able to lead relatively normal lives during the remission following the severe attack, and 3 were free of signs and symptoms almost all of the time during these long remissions. Eight of the group are still alive 7 years after the series study ended, increasing the longest period of life following the severe attacks to 25 years. Three of this group were first seen before 1949. Sixteen other patients lived 4 to 20 years after very severe attacks in which the severity on the arbitrary scale was grade 3. Ten of these have been able to lead quite normal lives and 6 have been free of signs and symptoms for long periods. Thirteen are still alive 7 years after the study ended, increasing the number who have lived 10 years or over after an attack of grade 3 activity to 12, with 7 alive more than 15 years after the attack. Inevitably, and probably advisedly, the majority of those of this group of 27 patients seen since 1949 were receiving steroids at the time of the severe attack. In 10 the steroid therapy was started 4 months to 12 years before the peak of the attack, but in 8 it was started at the time of the severe exacerbation. However, 5 patients who lived 6 to 23 years after being moribund received no steroids even with the attack and, similarly, 4 with severe attacks (grade 3 on the arbitrary scale) who lived 9 to 20 years after the attack received no steroids (cases 1 and 11, Appendix). Six of those 9 patients were treated at a time when steroids were available. It is thus apparent that steroid therapy cannot of itself always prevent exacerbations and that patients can recover from a moribund state with active lupus without the use of steroids. However, as has already been discussed, steroid therapy is usually indicated in patients in crisis, surely when severe hemolytic anemia or extreme thrombocytopenia is associated with the severe attack.

Exacerbations

The factors responsible for exacerbations are commonly apparent, and the aim of therapy during remissions is to avoid such factors if possible or, if not, to treat the exacerbation immediately with removal of the precipitating factor when possible and immediate resumption of the therapeutic regimen of physical and emotional rest, aspirin, and other drugs as indicated (see discussion under treatment).

Common precipitating factors are infection, followed by exacerbation in 85% (73 of 86) of the patients with infection in this series; physical and emotional stress, with exacerbation in 91% (41 of 45) in this series; pregnancy, with flare in 36% (27 of 82) in this series; operations, with flare in 23% (29 of 126) in this series; and exposure to sun or drugs such as sulfonamides and possibly hydralazine, tridione, diphenylhydantoin, and mephenytoin. In addition, ingestion of any drug to which the patient is allergic may lead to exacerbation.

Infection of any type and of almost any severity may cause exacerbation of lupus, whether the disease is in remission or active. Without doubt severe infections, most commonly respiratory, caused exacerbations that were often fatal in patients with or without active disease in the years before antibiotics were available. As has already been mentioned, the apparent onset of the disease was not uncommonly associated with severe infection, making it difficult to determine how much of the picture was due to lupus and how much to the infection. This same difficulty arises often now, especially in exacerbations, but the ability to control the infection in most cases has altered the subsequent course. However, infections remain one of the major precipitating factors in the apparent onset as well as in exacerbations of lupus and should be treated adequately with suitable antibiotics and with rest.

Physical and emotional stress are also major exacerbating factors. Overactivity may range from long hours of work, including heavy labor and housework; to house cleaning; to sports, including tennis, golf, swimming, skating, skiing, etc; to much dancing; to long walks; to traveling; to shoveling snow; to gardening; and to caring for sick members of the family. A much lesser degree of activity becomes stress to a patient whose disease is active, and may readily lead to exacerbation. Therefore, limitation of stresses to the extent that is possible becomes essential while the disease is still active.

Emotional stress may vary greatly in nature and degree, as would be expected. It may arise from one or a series of stressful situations, such as marital incompatibility, with or without divorce; alcoholism of spouse or a parent or a child; unemployment of self or spouse and loss of financial stability enhanced by medical expenses; lives of the older children and relatives that are unacceptable to the patient (including drugs, alcohol, illegitimate pregnancies, "unwise" marriages, incomplete education, etc); incompatible working conditions, especially in relation to those directly in charge of the patient's work, and lack of satisfaction in the work; retirement with its associated removal of many satisfactions and the altered home life; military service of any members of the immediate family; major decisions of any type, if difficult, including those related to change of job or of residence, or the attitude toward the children; demands of elderly parents, and guilt if the patient considers the attention given to the parents inadequate; difficult relationships with other members of the family such as siblings or those related to the patient by marriage.

Concern and worry, with or without justification, about any of these stresses, especially those related to the family or to the financial situation, may become major factors in causing exacerbation or in delaying, if not preventing, subsidence of the disease activity. Coupled with this, in many cases, is worry as to the outcome of the disease, with fear of crippling or death. Unfortunately, almost all material available to patients who try to "read about their disease" describes lupus as a fatal disease. This impression, while justified 20 years ago when 66% (36 of 54) died in 5 years, is not consistent with the fact that 57% (14 of 24) of the recent group of this series lived over 15 years. Anxiety and tension, presumably present before onset of the illness, are enhanced by the occurrence of the disease and, in some cases, may represent manifestations of SLE. Overreaction to many things results; to the symptoms of the disease itself; to the difficulty in accepting the limited life during the long period of active disease; to the attitude of others toward the disease or to the treatment that restricts the patient's activities so much even though she "looks so well"; to the necessity of choosing what activities to omit; to the guilty feeling because of inability to continue what she considers necessary, whether it be work at home and care of the family or work or other activities outside; and to the attempt to carry out the spouse's wishes and plans.

Associated with this combination of stresses is, in many patients, a more or less severe depression. This is often made worse by the frequently occurring depressive features caused by the disease and enhanced in some cases by steroid therapy. Treatment in this situation requires much of the physician's time and a real appreciation of the stresses.

Pregnancy commonly leads to exacerbation of SLE, as already discussed. The increased activity of disease may occur at any time from conception to 8 weeks or more after delivery. In our experience significant exacerbations occurred only in patients who had active disease at the time of pregnancy, and not in those whose disease had been in remission for many years (6 to 8). Therefore, while it is our impression that pregnancy is never entirely without danger in patients with SLE, if there seemed adequate reason for the patient to take the risk of pregnancy, we would recommend that it be delayed until the disease has been inactive for years (as will be discussed under treatment). Investigators vary in opinions on this decision.

Operations, both major and minor, may be followed by exacerbations of SLE in a day or two or at some time during the following few weeks. Even biopsies of the skin, muscle, lymph node, or kidney, or dental extractions may cause flares. It is apparent that all operative stress should be avoided if possible. Elective operations should be postponed until the activity of the disease is minimal. Procedures for diagnosis, prognosis, or determination of the course of the disease should be limited to those from which the results will add really significant evidence for diagnosis or will cause a sound basis for decisions as to therapy. Unnecessary support for the diagnosis, or a complete documentation of changes which can be considered with some certainty to be present, is inadvisable and adds to the risk of exacerbation or of delayed healing. When operative procedures of any type are necessary, precautions should be taken, as discussed in Chapter 5.

Exposure to sun may lead to varying degrees of exacerbation and should be avoided or protection as adequate as possible be used, as discussed under treatment. Known sensitivity to sun has been found in only one-third or less of patients with SLE, 34% (48 of 142) in this series, but it seems advisable to restrict sun exposure, at least to some extent, in all patients since overt sensitivity to sun may develop during the course of the disease.

The drugs that are generally accepted as exacerbating factors in SLE are sulfonamides. The exacerbations are usually severe and occasionally fatal. This group of drugs should not be used in lupus patients. Fortunately, their general use is relatively limited now but some forms, such as "gantrisin" (sulfisoxazole) are prescribed frequently and have caused flares of SLE in our experience. The groups of drugs that may produce syndromes indistinguishable from SLE should not be given to lupus patients if their use can be avoided. When one of the anticonvulsants has to be used, the dose should be as small as possible and reduced as rapidly as possible.

Exacerbation of SLE may occur upon withdrawal of any of the anti-inflammatory drugs used in therapy (see discussion in Chapter 5). In 3 patients in this series, exacerbation with recurrence of fever and joint

symptoms occurred in 48 hours after aspirin therapy was discontinued. The fever and symptoms subsided in 1 to 2 days after resumption
of aspirin. Exacerbation of SLE after withdrawal of corticosteroids is
seen frequently and always necessitates slow reduction in the dose.
Recently awareness of the possibility of exacerbation of SLE following
sudden withdrawal of azathioprine has increased. In a few patients
seen since this series ended we have noted such exacerbations.

The serious effect of a combination of stressful factors was seen in 1
of our patients who was allowed to go home for Christmas. On her
return following increased physical and emotional stress and the tem-
porary discontinuance of her steroid therapy, she was "almost moribund." She died on January 12.

Duration
The longest duration of disease from onset in the group first seen
before 1949 was approximately 50 years, the shortest 2½ months. The
longest duration from onset in the later series, first seen in 1949 or
since, was 26 years in a patient still alive now, making a total duration
of 33 years, and the shortest 7 months. The difficulty in determining
the exact onset of disease in some patients has already been discussed
and the method used in this series outlined.

From the first visit to the Massachusetts General Hospital, the longest duration was 43 years* and the shortest 1 day, in the group first
seen before 1949. In the later group the longest duration was 17 years
in patients still alive when the series was closed. Four of the patients
still alive when the series closed have lived 7 more years, making a
total duration of 24 years. The shortest duration in the group first seen
in 1949 or since was 2 weeks.

Duration from first visit showed significant correlation only with
sex. Twenty-seven percent of the females died in less than 12 months,
in contrast to 50% of the males. This difference probably reflects the
higher percentage of males in the group first seen before 1949, at a
time when the prognosis of the disease was not as good.

Survivorship
Survivorship in systemic lupus erythematosus, as calculated by the
method described in detail by Merrell and Shulman [164] has im-

---

*This patient was seen at the M.G.H. by the Dermatology Service in 1923, before
the present series was started, and was subsequently followed by us.

proved dramatically in the past 20 years (see Fig. 1). In the series of patients first seen before 1949, survivorship from the first visit was 34% (18 of 54) for 5 years and 24% (13) for 15 years, in contrast to 64% (15 of 24) for 5 years and 57% (14) for 15 years in the group seen since 1949 and also not treated with steroids. Unfortunately, this change in prognosis is not generally realized, although it has been reported also by other investigators [78, 128, 176, 220], and patients with lupus are still too frequently approached with the assumption that the life expectancy in the majority is less than 2 years. The effect of such an attitude on the handling of the patient is unfortunate, as will be discussed in Chapter 5. Any patient with SLE may live for many years, and it is impossible to determine the prognosis of any one case.

Comparison of survivorship in patients treated only with a "con-

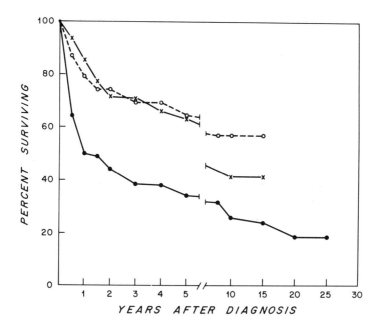

Figure 1. Survivorship after diagnosis of systemic lupus erythematosus. Percentages were calculated by the method described by Merrell and Shulman [176].

The solid circles (•) represent 54 patients first seen between 1923 and 1949 and treated conservatively. The open circles (O) represent 24 patients first seen in 1949 or later and treated conservatively. The crosses (X) represent 54 patients first seen in 1949 or later and treated with steroids.

servative" regime, as presented, with that in patients treated with steroids is extremely difficult. In the 54 patients in this series who received a significant degree of steroid therapy, the doses and duration of treatment varied markedly. (Seven patients who received only occasional doses over years or used some ointment were omitted, and also 7 patients who received short courses many years before death or in the week before death). The smallest dose at any one time was 5 mg per day and the highest 120 mg (except for 200 mg in 1 patient for 3 weeks) and duration varied from 1 month to 11 years. The estimated survivorships in the steroid and nonsteroid groups are quite similar (see Fig. 1), suggesting only a slightly increased survivorship in the steroid group in the first 18 months and a slightly decreased survivorship after 5 years. Whether these represent real differences cannot be determined.

In all of the survivorship curves (Fig. 1) it is apparent that mortality decreases significantly 2 to 3 years after the diagnosis is made, as demonstrated also by others [128, 173, 176]. When survivorship in the present series was calculated for the groups of patients in whom steroid therapy was started less than 2 years after onset or more than 2 years after onset, there was a significant difference (Fig. 2). The group in whom treatment was started early had a high mortality, especially in the first 2 years, and after 5 years. The other group had a moderately high mortality for less than 1 year and again after 5 years. The overall survivorship in the early group was 33% (12 of 37) after 15 years, in contrast to 56% (10 of 17) in the group in whom treatment was started more than 2 years after onset. Whether this indicates only that the patients in whom treatment was started early had more severe disease cannot be determined. The similar increase in percentage of survivorship after 2 years in the group treated "conservatively" suggests that other factors play a role.

In view of the large number of cases of SLE with relatively mild disease and the high percentage of survivorship, 57% for at least 15 years, the extremely pessimistic attitude of physicians and patients and all who deal with the patients is not justified. The likelihood of good remission is high and survival up to 40 years or more is possible. However, SLE remains a disease of possible sudden, severe, occasionally fatal exacerbations. These often lead to hasty and unwise therapy with anti-inflammatory agents of considerable potential toxicity, frequently associated with inadequate attention to the other important aspects of treatment.

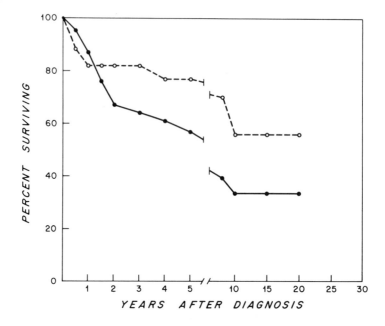

Figure 2. Survivorship after diagnosis of systemic lupus erythematosus in steroid-treated patients. The solid circles (•) represent the 37 patients in whom steroid treatment was started less than 2 years after onset. The open circles (O) represent the 17 patients in whom steroid treatment was started 2 years or more after onset.

Differences Between the Sexes

The disease is in general similar in males and females but differs slightly in some respects. The findings that showed significant differences are listed in Tables 5, 6, and 7.

The difference in age of onset (Table 5) has been reported in other series [69, 220]. However, the differences in other reports as to the predominance of males in children could not be evaluated in this series. There were only 12 patients under the age of 15 and none of them was male. Frequency of acute onset showed no significant difference between females (29%, 36 of 124) and males (39%, 7 of 18). The difference in the severity of the disease as determined by the number of episodes of greater than grade 3 activity was not great between males and females. However, a much higher percentage of males (55%, 10 of 18) than of females (23%, 29 of 124) died in the first episode of such severe activity. The course of the disease was steadily downhill in

Table 5. Comparison of clinical manifestations in 18 males and 124 females (except as indicated by notes).

Clinical manifestations	Observed in		Correlation p
	Male patients	Female patients	
"Typical" disease	69%	35%	0.025
Age of onset after 25	66	42	0.07
System first involved			
Facial rash	44	13	0.009
Systemic	6	27	
Intermittent arthritis	25	70	0.002
Morning stiffness	29[1]	77[2]	—
Hair loss	28	47	—
Vasomotor abnormalities	10	55	—
Diplopia	0	27	0.03
Psychosis	6	28	—
Convulsions	6	19	—
Elevated blood pressure	28	58	0.05
Subcutaneous nodules	12	21	—
Pericardial fluid	0	19	—
Rub	0	33	—
Systolic murmur $> 2/4$	0	19	—
Gallop	6	28	—

[1] Of 7 patients.
[2] Of 5 patients.

13% (16) of the 124 females, and 20% (4) of the 18 males (Table 7). These differences probably reflect, in part, the fact that a higher percentage of males (20%, 12 of 60) was present in the group seen before 1949, in contrast to 7% (6 of 82) in those seen in 1949 or later. Greater severity of disease and downhill course were found more commonly in the early group.

In summary, the significant differences are that males tend to have more "typical" disease; a slightly later age of onset; absence (in this series) of diplopia; a greater tendency toward facial rash as a presenting symptom, and less toward systemic involvement; a greatly re-

Table 6. Comparison of laboratory findings in 18 males and 124 females (except as indicated by notes).

Laboratory findings	Male patients	Female patients	Correlation p
Abnormal T waves	40%[1]	74%[2]	—
Increased PR interval	6	11	—
Abnormal liver-function tests	89[3]	62[4]	0.20
Abnormal number of red cells in urine	22	43	—
Hemoglobin			0.016
< 8 gm/100 ml	6	29	
< 6 gm/100 ml	0	9	
> 12 gm/100 ml always	61	40	
Coombs test positive	0[5]	30[6]	—
5% eosinophils or more	6	22	—
Splenomegaly at postmortem	100[7]	59[8]	0.01

[1] Of 10 patients.   [5] Of 5 patients.
[2] Of 97 patients.   [6] Of 53 patients.
[3] Of 9 patients.   [7] Of 9 patients.
[4] Of 77 patients.   [8] Of 49 patients.

duced incidence of psychoses; a markedly lessened tendency to have intermittent joint symptoms and morning stiffness; less elevation of blood pressure; greater tendency to enlargement of spleen; reduced clinical evidence of pericarditis; less tendency to have systolic murmur and gallop; a lessened incidence of vasomotor abnormalities; a less severe anemia; a reduced incidence of eosinophilia; a tendency to a lessened incidence of hematuria; and probably a slightly decreased tendency to have two or more remissions.

Table 7. Comparison of severity and course in 18 males and 124 females.

Severity and course	Male patients	Female patients	Correlation p
Death in 1st episode of > grade 3 activity	55%	23%	—
Steadily downhill course	20	13	0.13
Two or more remissions	17	49	—
Duration from 1st visit < 12 months	50	29	—

Differences Before and After 1949

A decrease in the severity of systemic lupus erythematosus over the past 20 to 25 years has been clearly demonstrated both by us (see Fig. 1) and by others. As discussed above, all of the reasons for the difference are not known. In addition to the definite decrease in mortality, changes in the manifestations and course of the disease in the past 20 to 25 years were found in our series, as shown in Tables 8 and 9.

Outstanding in the altered manifestations were the increased incidence of renal disease and psychoses in the later group, as noted by others. Coincidentally there was also increase in involvement of joints but decrease in the presence of butterfly rash.

Striking in the group first seen before 1949 was the high incidence of acute disease with steadily downhill course and death within 1 year from onset. In the later group this course had become unusual.

Causes of Death

It is often difficult in SLE to ascribe death to a single cause, since so many systems are involved and the abnormality in several different

Table 8. Comparison of manifestations in 60 patients first seen before 1949 with those in 82 patients first seen in 1949 or later.

| Manifestations | Patients first seen | | Correlation p |
	Before 1949 (60)	In 1949 or later (82)	
Acute onset	82%	59%	0.005
System involved			
Joints	21	38	0.07
Skin	25	13	0.07
No joint involvement	25	6	0.005
Psychosis (without steroid therapy)	17	37	0.009
Elevated NPN or BUN	31	57	0.007
Abnormal number of red cells in urine	27	52	0.004
Many casts	19	38	0.05
No casts	40	27	—
Butterfly rash	90	73	—

Table 9. Comparison of course and severity in 60 patients first seen before 1949 with those in 82 patients first seen in 1949 or later.

Course and severity	Patients first seen		
	Before 1949 (60)	In 1949 or later (82)	Correlation p
Steadily downhill	25%	7%	0.005
Two or more remissions	28	55	—
Only 1 episode of > grade 3			
Terminal	47	16	< 0.001
With recovery	8	22	—
Two episodes of > grade 3	30	44	—
Duration from first visit			
< 1 yr.	47	21	< 0.001
3 yrs. or more	38	59	—
Duration from onset			
< 1 yr.	32	5	< 0.001
3 yrs. or more	48	77	—

systems is often adequate in itself to produce death. However, classification has been attempted in this series, especially in the effort to determine in what percentage of patients the renal disease played a significant role in the death.

Of the 60 patients first seen before 1949, 11 were still alive when the series ended, 43 had died, and 6 were lost. In the later group of 82 patients, 41 were still alive, 39 had died, and 2 were lost.

A major cause of death in the series of patients first seen before 1949 was active lupus, as found in 17 patients (40% of 43) (see Table 10). Ten of these had no one specific severe localization of the disease, whereas 3 had predominantly serositis, 2 myocarditis with cardiac failure, 1 severe liver disease and colitis, and 1 cerebral hemorrhage presumably resulting from lupus involvement of the central nervous system. Renal function as indicated by urine analysis or levels of NPN or BUN in the serum was normal in this group, except in 3 patients in whom the NPN levels were 42, 50, and 88 mg/100 ml. The latter level occurred terminally in 1 of the patients with cardiac failure. Corroboration of the fact that renal disease played little or no role in the death of this group of patients was obtained at postmortem examination. In

Table 10. Causes of death in the 82 patients who died.

Causes of death	In 43 patients first seen before 1949		In 39 patients first seen in 1949 or later	
	Number	Number in whom renal involvement played little or no role in death	Number	Number in whom renal involvement played little or no role in death
Active SLE				
no specific localization	10	10	3	3
serositis predominant	3	1	1	1
myocarditis	2	1	3	2
colitis and liver involvement	1	1	0	0
central nervous system involvement	1 (CVA)	1	7 (2 CVA)	5
Infection with active SLE	17	15	8	7
GI hemorrhage	2	2	1	0
Uremia	6	0	14	0
Cor pulmonale	0	0	1	1
10 hours postvalvulotomy	0	0	1	1
Myocardial infarction	1	0	0	0
	43	31	39	20

the 11 patients on whom autopsies were performed, the glomeruli were negative by light microscopy in 4 cases and showed rare hyalinization, or focal basement membrane thickening, or a few focal accumulations of polymorphonuclears, or focal areas of necrosis in 1 or more tufts in the other 7 patients. In the patient with NPN level of 50 mg, these foci of necrosis in 1 or more tufts involved most glomeruli.

An equally common cause of death in the early series was infection, usually associated, of course, with exacerbation of the lupus activity. As noted above, it was generally difficult to determine how much of the clinical picture was due to the infection and how much to the active SLE. Infection was the major cause in 17 patients of 43 (40%). In this group renal function as indicated by urine analysis or NPN or BUN levels in the serum was normal in all except 5 patients. In 4 the terminal NPN levels were 45, 47, 64, and 84 mg/100 ml, the latter occurring in a patient who had cardiac failure. The fifth patient had mild nephrosis with a serum albumin of 3.0 gm and an NPN of 48 mg. The relatively slight degree of renal involvement in the group that died of infection was clearly demonstrated at postmortem examinations. In the 16 patients on whom autopsies were performed the glomeruli were negative in 4 cases, showed congestion of capillary tufts in 1, some wire loops in 2, and focal necrosis in single loops or parts of loops in 6, varying in distribution from usually occasional glomeruli to the majority in 1 case. The glomeruli in the patient with the NPN level of 64 mg per 100 ml showed occasional areas suggesting wire loops, a few areas of fibrinoid necrosis, and occasional areas of lymphocytic infiltration with fibrosed glomeruli. In the patient with the terminal serum NPN level of 84 mg/100 ml, the glomeruli were slightly cellular and there were eosinophilic hyaline deposits around the basement membrane. The glomeruli in the patient with nephrosis showed widespread patchy focal necrosis with some infiltration. In 2 patients with septicemia the kidneys showed focal areas of polymorphonuclear infiltration. Factors presumably related to the activity of SLE played a major role in 2 of the patients who died from infection, 1 of whom had a cerebral hemorrhage, and 1 had terminal seizures.

Two other patients died after severe hemorrhages, one gastrointestinal and one epistaxis. One of these patients had moderate albuminuria but at postmortem examination the glomeruli were negative except for rare replacement by scars.

In this group of patients first seen before 1949, only 6 patients of 43 (14%) died of uremia. This is a slightly lower incidence than found by Stickney and Keith [255]. The sera showed levels of 90 to 100 mg/100 ml as NPN and 55 and 152 mg as BUN. Many factors other than renal failure were present in the patient with the BUN level of 55 mg/ml. He had had an exacerbation of SLE, followed by a severe respiratory infection, for which he had been given sulfonamides.

One patient died after a myocardial infarction. Postmortem examination showed severe atherosclerosis of coronary arteries and the interlobular and arcuate renal vessels. The glomeruli showed some fibrinoid swelling, moderate exudate, and slight proliferation.

It is thus apparent that renal disease played relatively little or no role in the death of approximately 72% (31) of the 43 patients in the early series. In another 12% (5) it probably played only a small role.

In the later series of patients, first seen in 1949 or since, the relative proportions of the causes of death showed great variation from that in the early series (see Table 10). Deaths from active lupus had decreased only from 40% of 43 to 36% of 39 but the distribution was different. Of the 14 patients in this group who died of active lupus, 3 had no specific severe localization, 1 had predominantly serositis, 3 myocarditis, and 7 had central nervous system involvement. In contrast to the findings in the series of patients first seen before 1949, there were 4 patients in the later series who died of seizures, 1 of suicide, and 2 of cerebral hemorrhage. In only 1 of the patients with seizures the NPN level was abnormal, 67 mg/100 ml. Postmortem examinations were performed on 2 of the patients with seizures. Some glomeruli showed minimal areas of fibrinoid necrosis in 1, and in the other patient in whom the NPN level was 67 mg/100 ml there were some crescents, some thickening of the basement membrane, and many fibrotic glomeruli. Renal function as indicated by urine analysis and/or levels of NPN and BUN in the serum was normal in the other patients in this group with active lupus, except in 2 patients with cardiac failure in whom the terminal NPN levels were 50 and 78 mg/100 ml. The absence of significant renal involvement was corroborated in the 5 patients on whom postmortem examinations were performed. The glomeruli were negative in 1 patient and showed minimal focal changes in 3 others, including the patient with NPN level of 50 mg/100 ml, with slight infiltration or some wire loops, or a few crescents or rare hematoxylin bodies or some hyalinization. In the patient with a terminal NPN level of 78 mg/100 ml the kidney showed cellular infiltration in some glomeruli, scattered crescents, and prominent wire loops. Cardiac arrest occurred during surgery for probable tamponade in one of this group of patients. In view of our present knowledge of the more favorable course of the disease, it is of significance that attempts at resuscitation were less strenuous than usual, partly because of the poor prognosis in SLE generally assumed at that time.

Infection, which was the major cause of death in the early series, had fallen in incidence in the group seen in 1949 or later from 40% to 21%. This is certainly attributable to the availability of effective antibiotics. In the majority of these patients in whom infection was the major cause of death, it was associated with exacerbation of the activity of the lupus. Five of the 8 patients who died of infection were receiving steroids, ranging in dose from 30 to 60 mg of prednisone or the equivalent. Urine analysis and/or serum levels of NPN or BUN indicated normal renal function except in 3 patients; in 2 of these the NPN levels were 56 and 64 mg/100 ml, and in the third the BUN level was 30 mg/100 ml. Corroboration of relatively mild renal involvement was obtained at postmortem examinations, which were performed in all of the group. The glomeruli were negative in 1 patient and in 6 others showed focal areas of thickening of the basement membrane, or rare fibrinoid, or some crescents. In the eighth patient, in whom the NPN level was 64 mg/100 ml, there were moderate to marked wire loops and rare areas of necrosis of tufts. Presumably the activity of SLE played a role in the immediate cause of death of 2 of these patients, 1 of whom had seizures with cardiac arrest and 1 had cardiac failure.

Severe gastrointestinal hemorrhage was the cause of death in 1 patient. The NPN was 31 mg/100 ml. Postmortem examination was not performed in this case. The percentage of patients dying of gastro-intestinal hemorrhage was essentially the same in the early and the late series.

One patient died of cor pulmonale after 17 years of disease. Renal function by clinical tests was normal and at postmortem examination the glomeruli showed only scattered foci of lymphocytes.

Another patient died 10 hours after valvuloplasty. Urine analyses were normal and the BUN level was 37 mg/100 ml. At autopsy, the glomeruli showed congestion with occasional foci of infiltration and occasional periglomerular fibrosis.

In contrast to the series of patients seen before 1949, renal disease played relatively little or no role in the death of only 51% (20 of 39) instead of 72% (31 of 43) of the patients. In another 10% (4) it prob-ably played only a small role. It is of great interest that the percentage of patients dying of renal failure had risen from 14% (6 of 43) to 36% (14 of 39), an incidence somewhat lower than that in the series of Cook [55], Muehrcke et al. [187], and Cheatum et al. [47], but com-parable to that of Rothfield et al. [214] and Copeland et al. [57]. In the 14 patients in whom renal failure was the major cause of death, the serum showed NPN levels of 110 and 137 mg/100 ml in 3 patients and the BUN levels in the other 11 patients ranged from 95 to 270 mg/100 ml.

Factors other than renal failure also played major roles in the pa-tients with renal failure. The immediate cause of death in one of these patients was septicemia with Gram-negative bacilli; in another, severe gastrointestinal bleeding and pneumonia; in another, a cerebral hem-orrhage, and in 2 others, terminal seizures. One of the latter occurred in the patient who had had renal infarcts.

The reason for the increased number of patients dying of renal fail-ure in the group first seen in 1949 or later is not apparent. Frequently it is argued that the ability to keep the patients alive a longer period of time with the use of antibiotics and corticosteroids allows the renal disease to progress to become a major manifestation. Of the 11 patients in the present series who showed no glomerular changes at post-mortem examination, 8 were first seen before 1949. Of these, 5 died in less than 2 years and the other 3 in severe exacerbations after several years of mild disease. It is of interest also that significant and often fatal involvement of the central nervous system has become more common during the same period since 1949, as indicated also by the study of Cheatum et al. [47].

5 Treatment

Evaluation of Treatment

In a disease in which the course is so varied and the time of occurrence of exacerbations or remissions so unpredictable, evaluation of the effect of treatment is extremely difficult and often impossible. Further problems in judging the results of therapy in many series arise from the lack of any proof of the diagnosis and from the absence of generally accepted criteria. There is a tendency, therefore, for different types of patients to be included in various series and for the degree of activity of the disease and the extent of involvement to differ for this reason. As a result, comparison often cannot be made among the reports from different investigators. Statements as to the effect of any treatment in a series of patients apply only to other patients selected by the same criteria.

A major difficulty in the evaluation of treatment in SLE is the fact that a random selection double-blind study with adequate follow-up has never been done and perhaps never can be done in proper fashion because of the possibility of the occurrence of "lupus crisis" or other life-threatening complications which would necessitate breaking the assigned treatment regimen. It is apparent that there is as yet no "cure," and no "proof" of the value of any therapeutic regimen in systemic lupus erythematosus. Only empirical impressions from relatively large series of patients diagnosed by well-defined criteria and followed for several years, at least, can be helpful in determining the choice of treatment. Of relatively little value are uncontrolled, short-term (2 to 6 months) studies of therapeutic agents, with conclusions as to the value of the medication drawn from slight to moderate clinical changes. This is especially true if changes are hard to interpret, such as minor change in creatinine clearance despite some lowering of the serum creatinine. The effect of such studies may be only to give unjustified support for a toxic medication and encourage physicians to emphasize such medications at the expense of other aspects of a good therapeutic regimen. Notorious in SLE is the inability of any physician to foresee the course in any patient, whatever medication is used. In many cases the natural course of the disease with good conservative therapy is comparable to results that might be ascribed to specific medications. The similarity is indicated by the comparable survivorship in the patients of this series first seen in 1949 or since and all treated conservatively, and in the series reported by Merrell and Shulman [176] in which 75% of the patients received steroids (see Fig. 1). Equally unwise is a tendency to consider marked improvement for less than 1 month as a remission. If the percentage of remissions is calculated, it should include separate groups for those of short (1 to 3 months), medium (3 months to 3 years) and long duration (over 3 years).

"Conservative" Regimen

Rest

A basic regimen of physical and emotional rest would be recommended by many physicians active in the treatment of patients with SLE, despite the absence of any proof of its value. The difficulty in evaluating the effect of any treatment and the inability to determine the therapeutic effect of rest when it is part of a complete regimen make proof of the value of rest impossible. Only empirical evidence from large series of patients can be used. From my experience it is my opinion that complete bed rest is indicated during periods of really active disease with such symptoms as marked weakness and fatiguability, headache, chest pain, abdominal pain, severe emotional disturbance, or marked joint pains; and with such signs as fever, acute typical rash, pleural or pericardial rub, edema, swollen tender joints, or psychosis, along with laboratory evidence of great activity such as severe anemia, marked leukopenia, thrombocytopenia, albuminuria, hematuria, elevated sedimentation rate, or low complement levels. The decision as to whether or not any ambulation, even lavatory privileges, should be allowed varies more. When weakness and fatiguability are great, the simple process of getting up even to use a commode near the bed often represents a real effort, recognized as such by the patient, and in at least 15 cases improvement has appeared to be faster when complete bed rest was resumed. A period when rest is often grossly neglected is that of the first 24 hours after admission when the patient may be very ill. During that period, several episodes of history-taking and physical, neurological, and psychological examination, in addition to many often strenuous tests, may cause extreme fatigue and in some cases, apparently, increased exacerbation of the disease. Many patients complain that they are "very tired" after such a process.

When the disease is less active, the amount of bed rest required varies with the severity. In general, patients with SLE need bed rest for at least 20 hours a day for many months after a severe attack. It should be continued until the marked fatiguability has disappeared and all symptoms and signs have become minor, and until the hemoglobin and platelets have improved markedly, the hematuria subsided, and the creatinine clearance returned to a constant level. Physical activity can then be increased slowly, with immediate return to the preceding level if symptoms, signs, or laboratory findings worsen. Some degree of rest greater than that obtained by most people, usually 12 hours or more, should be taken by lupus patients for many years after a period of active disease. Haserick [103] suggests that children should not return to school for 1 year after an acute phase. Patients who have lupus remain "fragile" and susceptible to exacerbations for years, as reported also by others [184]. It appears from our series that this "fragility" lessens continuously but slowly during periods of remission. Perhaps the patients never become able to stand excessive stresses but some at least can finally withstand pregnancy, marked physical and emotional disturbances, and infections without exacerbation of the lupus.

Treatment of Psychogenic Factors

Emotional rest, of importance as great as or possibly greater than physical rest, is much harder to obtain and a great deal more of the physician's time is required to aid in achieving it. The emotional factors are numerous. In the majority of patients psychogenic factors, often of environmental nature, have played a role in precipitating the attack in 90% (41 of 45) in this series, and usually remain and disturb the patients, often to a major degree. These must be considered and help given in the handling of them to the extent possible. Supportive psychiatric treatment is often of great assistance at this stage and throughout the attack.

Fear of the disease, especially of the severe manifestations of "crisis" or of death, is a major factor in some patients. In all cases, but especially in this group, great reassurance is necessary. Far too often the patients know the name "lupus" and almost invariably have heard a dramatic but incorrect labelling of it as a rapidly fatal disease. Direct and indirect reference to the high percentage of patients who go into remission and live many years may help. Unsolicited statements as to things a patient will be doing "later" or "next year" are often of some value. Additional psychogenic elements may arise from the disease itself, presumably from vasculitis involving cerebral vessels, as interpreted by others [62, 86, 165, 194]. These subside as the disease goes into remission and need no special treatment. There is no proof that steroid therapy is of specific value in treatment of the lupus psychoses. Few cases suggesting specific value of steroids have been reported. To be sure, if the patient is severely ill and the disease in "crisis," steroid therapy may be necessary to control the exacerbation and, concomitantly, the psychotic manifestations may subside. Not uncommonly, however, the psychotic manifestations subside very slowly so that it may be 1 to 2 years or even more before the patient is normal psychologically. In our experience the improvement continues despite slow withdrawal of steroid therapy when the "crisis" has subsided. Still another element in the psychological disturbances in SLE may be the reaction to corticosteroids. This may take as many forms as the manifestations of the disease and is often hard to differentiate (as described above). Therapy consists of the withdrawal of the steroids as rapidly as can be done without exacerbation.

Often throughout the psychoses of lupus, a moderate degree of insight persists and dread of "being crazy" is added to the other fears and must be considered in the handling of the patient, requiring reassurance and sometimes belittling of the psychiatric abnormality. During the long period of convalescence, frustration from the limitations imposed by the fatigue and other symptoms of the disease and from the enforced rest may be great. The physician's optimism, which is essential for assisting the patient at this stage, is legitimate, being based on the high tendency of the disease to remit and the relatively low mortality now as compared with 25 years ago. Such knowledge and optimism transmitted to the patient is in my opinion of importance as great as or greater than the persistent use of high doses of any anti-inflammatory drugs. A similar attitude was expressed by Hill [109], who stated that "a Gladstonian air of expectancy may well be more rewarding than the most energetic use of powerful hormones."

Convulsions, which do not necessarily occur in the patients who have psychoses, often are of serious import. Almost half of the patients with seizures in our series had them only in the terminal episode. There is no evidence that steroid therapy alters the incidence. Diphenylhydantoin in doses from 100 to 300 mg as indicated is usually given, though it is difficult to determine its effect. Caution should be taken not to continue this drug longer than seems essential, since a few exacerbations of the disease probably enhanced by diphenylhydantoin have been reported [3]. In our patients, 3 had mild exacerbations soon after such therapy was started and appeared to improve again with discontinuance of the diphenylhydantoin. Symptomatic treatment during the convulsions is indicated, of course, and it is our opinion that oxygen should be given since at least 2 of our patients became extremely anoxic after the seizures and succumbed.

Diet

No specific diet is indicated in SLE unless renal insufficiency requires limitation of protein, nephrosis or steroid therapy requires limitation of sodium, or the weight of the patient indicates a higher or lower caloric intake. High doses of corticosteroids may necessitate increased intake of potassium. When indicated by low blood levels of iron and a persistently low hemoglobin concentration, ferrous salts should be given. If the hematocrit does not rise with improving disease and no iron lack is found, transfusions can often be of value.

Transfusions

The value of transfusions is not generally realized. In our experience there has been a suggestion that transfusions have a therapeutic value even above any effect on hemoglobin levels. In many patients of this series with severe, active disease, especially those seen before corticosteroids were available, transfusions were given every 2 to 3 days and continued even after hemoglobin had risen to 12 gm/100 ml or more. Such treatment was associated with improvement in at least 20 cases, but, as with most of the therapeutic measures discussed, it was impossible to be sure what role the transfusion played. In this series there has been no obvious reaction to transfusions, but because of this possibility the use of frozen washed red cells has been suggested. The hemoglobin level usually rises significantly after transfusion, but frequently does not rise further until the disease activity decreases or another transfusion is given. In such cases elevated reticulocyte counts often indicate persistence of hemolysis. The urobilinogen concentration may not be high and the Coombs test may or may not be positive. Apparently the rate of production of red cells and the rate of hemolysis are in equilibrium and remain so even when the hematocrit has been increased by transfusion. The fact that the higher level can be maintained may again suggest that the transfusion has lessened the activity of the disease to some extent.

Treatment of Infections

Of utmost importance in the treatment of SLE is control of infections. All identified organisms should, of course, be treated adequately with suitable antibiotics. Exceptional danger of sensitivity need not be feared, except in the case of sulfonamides, which should never be used in SLE. Despite occasional references to sensitivity of SLE patients to penicillin [69, 146], it has not been apparent in our experience, being present in only 2%. In many cases of lupus in crisis it is impossible to tell how much of the picture is due to the activity of SLE and how much to an accompanying infection. In such patients it is often advisable to treat with a broad-spectrum antibiotic even before the results of cultures are known or in the presence of negative cultures.

Protection from Sun Exposure

Protection from ultraviolet rays of the sun is often of great value and can now be accomplished to a considerable degree by the use of sun shields such as sulisobenzone or para-aminobenzoic acid. In addition, it is safest to recommend that all patients with SLE always avoid direct exposure to the sun and wear hats with brims and clothes that cover as much of the body as possible when any extended sun exposure is likely. It is our belief that all the means of protection should be used in all patients even though only 20% are sensitive. Sun sensitivity may develop during the course of the disease.

Pregnancy

Pregnancy should be avoided in patients with SLE, at least while the disease is active or severe renal disease is present, as recommended also by Rothfield [212]. In making this recommendation to the patient and her husband or fiancé it is wise to emphasize the increased likelihood of miscarriage and the real danger of exacerbation of SLE which could be severe. At the same time, the lessened danger from pregnancy after the disease has become inactive should be strongly emphasized. If the patient has persistent renal disease, pregnancy should be avoided even if the disease seems inactive otherwise. In many cases, adoption may be the wisest procedure. It is not advisable to use hormones for contraception since their use has been followed by increased activity of SLE in a few patients, both in our experience and that of others [139]. Premature interruption of pregnancy after the first 6 weeks should not usually be recommended since exacerbation of lupus has been reported to occur almost as frequently then as after full-term deliveries [69]. After delivery, whether at term or prematurely, attempts should be made to lessen the likelihood of exacerbation. Stresses should be avoided to the extent possible. It is desirable for the patient to remain in the hospital for 1 or 2 extra days and then have full help at home for at least a week, and some household help for at least a month. Breast feeding should be avoided.

Operations

Operations of any type may cause exacerbation of SLE. If elective, they should be postponed until the activity of lupus subsides. If an operation is necessary, the patient should be kept in the hospital, with many hours of rest daily, for several more days postoperatively than the specific type of operation would usually require. Convalescence should be prolonged until fatiguability has decreased at least to the preoperative level. Hospitalization is usually advisable even for minor procedures such as extraction of teeth. Sympathectomy for finger or toe ulcerations or vasomotor symptoms alone is usually contraindicated, not only because of the real danger of exacerbation of the lupus as with other operations, but also because of the likelihood that the vasomotor symptoms and the ulcerations will not subside postoperatively or, if they do, will recur within months. The ulcerations are best treated with complete bed rest and the use of reserpine, dibenzylin, or tolazoline. Reserpine may be effective orally in doses up to 0.25 mg t.i.d. or q.i.d. if tolerated. Splenectomy should be avoided if possible because of the potential exacerbation of SLE [63, 120]. However, it may be necessary if the platelet count remains at a bleeding level (below 10,000 per cu mm) after full treatment including corticosteroid administration. In 1 patient of this series, the platelet count remained low (4,000 per cu mm) on steroid therapy. Splenectomy was performed. The platelet count rose but could not be maintained at an adequate level without continued steroid therapy. In this case, the operation had merely made the steroid therapy effective in maintaining the platelet level, as found by others [57, 69].

Surgical treatment of acute abdominal episodes, such as appendicitis or cholecystitis with stones in the ducts, is essential. However, in many cases it is extremely difficult to differentiate these acute surgical emergencies from peritonitis and vasculitis due to active SLE. The physical and laboratory findings may be identical. Operation should be avoided, if possible, but the patient must be observed very closely to note any definite indications of a surgical emergency. Peritoneal aspiration was of diagnostic value in one of the cases in this series. Further difficulty in this ominous situation is the ability of corticosteroid therapy to lessen or remove the physical manifestations of an acute abdominal crisis.

Anti-inflammatory Drugs

In addition to the essential basic conservative regimen used for all patients, anti-inflammatory drugs should be given. There are strong differences of opinion as to which of these agents to use at any one time and for what period the use should be continued. As has already been discussed, there is insufficient evidence on which to base these decisions, despite some statements to the contrary in the literature, and only the experience of investigators with groups of patients classified by strict criteria and followed for several years at least can be of help. The three groups of agents most commonly used and most discussed are salicylates, corticosteroids, and cytotoxic drugs.

Aspirin

Administration of aspirin is considered by many physicians to be part of the "basic regimen" for all patients with systemic lupus erythematosus and I think its use is advisable in all patients if possible. Other investigators would limit its use to those patients who have joint or muscle symptoms. This is not wise. There seems little question but that the anti-inflammatory effect of aspirin, in some cases at least, extends beyond the joints, as one might expect from the demonstration of its anti-inflammatory potency in the lesions caused by silver nitrate in tissues [143]. In our series, severe exacerbations with increase in fever, redness, and joint pains followed withdrawal of aspirin (as had, in a few cases, been predicted by me) and these subsided within hours with reinstitution of the medication. These cases seem to indicate a more general anti-inflammatory effect. The intriguing question as to its value in renal inflammation is unanswered, as with steroids and azathioprine, and will remain so unless a proper random-selection, blindfold study can be made.

Recent studies of the comparative anti-inflammatory effect of acetylsalicylic acid and sodium salicylate show a greater reduction of inflammation with aspirin [74]. This is in accord with the clinical impression obtained by us and others [54] in the treatment of patients with rheumatoid arthritis. As a result we have used aspirin, not sodium salicylate, for our patients with SLE.

Clinical experience suggests that a full dose, producing blood levels just below toxicity, is most effective. The apparent improvement in at least 20 patients in our experience when low blood levels have been raised to such concentrations supports this thesis. Studies in this laboratory [209] have indicated that the toxic salicylate level varies greatly with age. In children below the age of 10, toxicity is rarely, if ever, encountered with blood levels of 40 mg /100 ml or less. From the age of 11 to 20 the toxic level is usually about 35 to 40 mg, and from the age of 21 to 65 this level is between 25 and 30 mg/100 ml. Above the age of 65 the concentration must usually be between 15 and 20 mg to avoid toxicity. Therefore, therapeutic levels should be, in general, those indicated in Table 11.

In most patients above the age of 15 it is not necessary to determine salicylate levels, since the toxic level can be recognized by increasing the dose until persistent tinnitus or slight deafness is produced. The dose should then be reduced by 0.6 gm and maintained steadily at that level. It is essential to appreciate the difference in blood levels produced in different individuals by the same number of aspirin tablets. The dose should never be a routine number of tablets, such as the

Table 11. Desirable therapeutic levels of aspirin.

Age	Concentration of salicylate/100 ml
< 10 years	35-40 mg
11 to 20	30-35 mg
21 to 65	25-30 mg
> 65	15-20 mg

almost universally recommended 8 300-mg tablets a day, but rather the amount that will produce a concentration just below toxicity, determined as described above. In our studies, 8 tablets a day gave salicylate levels varying from 8 to 40 mg/100 ml in patients between the ages of 15 and 65 [209]. The differences did not correlate with the weight of the individuals. It is thus apparent that there is no standard number of tablets for all patients and the number must be determined for each person. Commonly, in patients between the ages of 15 and 60, it is advisable to start with a reasonable number, such as 3 tablets four times a day, and increase as is usually necessary to reach the desired level. In young children it is usually necessary to determine the salicylate level at least once, to establish the dose. While children are under observation in a hospital, the concentration can be maintained safely at 40 mg/100 ml, but at home a level of about 35 mg/100 ml is preferable since fever, gastrointestinal disturbances and dehydration, or other illness may cause rapid changes to toxic levels.

Aspirin should be continued until remission has occurred, and this is possible in view of the relatively slight toxicity. When symptoms and signs have subsided and laboratory determinations have returned to normal, with the possible exception of a slight persistent elevation of sedimentation rate or positive LE cell test or slight albuminuria of constant amount, the dose of aspirin can be reduced slowly. Withdrawal of ¼ of the dose for the first 1 or 2 months and then similar reductions every 1 or 2 months will usually not be followed by any apparent exacerbation. Full dosage should be resumed if symptoms or signs recur at that time or later.

The recognized toxicity of aspirin at therapeutic levels is not great. Most troublesome is the gastrointestinal irritation that may occur. The incidence of this is not known since protected forms of aspirin tablets are so generally prescribed, but, before such were available, it was our impression that perhaps 10 to 20% of patients had significant gastric symptoms. In studies of the loss of blood from the gastrointestinal tract on 1,500-mg doses of aspirin a day, it has been demonstrated that an average of 4 ml per day may be lost [281]. That this significantly affects the hemoglobin concentration or iron level has not been demonstrated. The loss has been shown to decrease in a few days [54]. In practice, if gastric symptoms are produced by aspirin, they can be prevented usually by use of one of the many available protected forms of tablets made with either a buffering mixture or an enteric coating. With the use of coated tablets it is necessary to be sure, by deafness, tinnitus, or salicylate levels, that absorption is adequate. Further protection is occasionally necessary as provided by ingestion of the aspirin with food, especially milk, and by simultaneous use of additional buffers containing aluminum hydroxide. Rarely a six-meal diet is necessary. Very rarely gross gastric bleeding may occur, but there is still no evidence that aspirin causes peptic ulceration [54]. In fact, with the above regimen, patients with known peptic ulcers, with or without bleeding, can usually take aspirin without difficulty.

A common evidence of definite aspirin toxicity is deafness. This is not of serious import and has been shown to subside with removal of the medicine in humans even after years of slight deafness [189], and in experimental monkeys [190]. Detailed study showed no histological damage in the monkeys. Rarely a patient, usually 50 years of age or older, may develop troublesome tinnitus on a relatively small dose of aspirin and it becomes impossible to increase the dosage to adequate levels.

Significant increase in prothrombin time with bleeding is not found with therapeutic levels of aspirin except when liver disease of moderate degree is present. Clinically insignificant increases have been reported occasionally since the early studies in 1940. Aspirin can be given to patients receiving anticoagulants, but the dose of anticoagulant may have to be reduced and the aspirin dosage kept slightly below the usual level. Careful monitoring is necessary. Furthermore, aspirin should be given with great caution if a patient has decreased liver function. In our experience the prothrombin time may become markedly prolonged and bleeding may ensue.

The reduced adhesiveness of platelets in the presence of aspirin has been well demonstrated [257], but the frequency of any effect on bleeding in patients without a bleeding diathesis is not yet known. Even patients with SLE treated with aspirin have not usually had any bleeding except in the presence of thrombocytopenia or local areas of vascultis. Whether the very rare instance of unexplained bleeding is related to the effect of aspirin on platelet adhesiveness is not known.

The many other physiologic alterations produced by aspirin, including the effect on thyroid activity and on pulmonary function [54], have not been related to clinical effects of therapeutic doses of aspirin, at least in adults.

Corticosteroids

Corticosteroids, which are commonly used in the therapy of patients with SLE, have much greater and more rapid anti-inflammatory effects than aspirin but also much greater toxicity. There persists great difference of opinion as to what clinical picture and laboratory findings indicate a need for steroid treatment. Obviously when a patient is in "lupus crisis" or unquestionably dangerously ill, steroids would be given by all physicians, the only question being the dose, which will be discussed below. Similarly, when severe hemolytic anemia (hematocrit less than 20) or thrombocytopenia (platelet count less than 50,000/cu mm) is present, even without other serious signs, steroid therapy is indicated. There are few, if any, other organ system involvements that have been shown by adequate studies to require steroid therapy or to have a better course in long-time follow-up with such therapy. In my experience corticosteroids are rarely necessary in any patients except those severely ill or in crisis, or with severe hemolytic anemia or thrombocytopenia. Despite this fact, many physicians give steroids to every patient in whom a diagnosis of SLE is made, even though the diagnosis in some cases rests largely on the finding of an LE cell. This is bad treatment.

In the present series only 72% (58) of the 82 patients first seen in 1949 or since have ever received any steroids, except for 9 patients who received occasional doses or used some ointment. Emphasis on the fact that steroid therapy is not necessary in all cases of SLE is given by the fact that 57% (14) of the 24 patients seen in 1949 or since who received no steroids lived 15 years or more from the first visit to M.G.H., in contrast to 41% (24) of the 58 on steroid therapy. The group who received no steroids may have had slightly less severe disease than those treated with steroids, but it included many severe cases.

Usually, of course, with the treatment of any SLE patient with steroids there is a rapid improvement in sense of well-being and appetite and often in hemoglobin, and a decrease in the relatively nonserious manifestations of the disease, such as fever, serositis, and joint pains (including pain of chest wall origin). Occasionally even on a dose of 40 mg or more of prednisone, joint pains persist and require aspirin for control. However, inherent in steroid therapy are the many potential toxic manifestations of the drugs so well known to all physicians. With high doses of steroids the loss of potassium and the retention of sodium necessitate an increased intake of potassium and decreased intake of sodium. In all patients who have ever had tuberculosis or have evidence in chest x-ray, isoniazid should be given throughout the course of steroid therapy. Of even greater concern than the toxicity is the difficulty in withdrawing the medication. Since the effect of corticosteroid therapy is merely suppression of the inflammation and not "healing" or "removal" of the underlying cause, withdrawal of the steroids often allows recurrence of the inflammation and the associated symptoms and signs. In 2 patients of this series death occurred within 2 weeks of rapid withdrawal. In most cases the exacerbation can be avoided or greatly reduced by very slow reduction in the dose over the course of a year or two if necessary, as described below. However, the necessity for such slow reduction brings further difficulty by prolonging the period of time the patient is on treatment and increasing the severity of associated "toxicity," of great seriousness being the increased susceptibility to infection with late recognition and poor handling, and the loss of calcium from vertebrae and other bones. In severe cases it may not be possible to withdraw steroids completely.

Survivorship in the series of 24 patients first seen in 1949 or since (Fig. 1) and treated with the conservative regime is quite comparable to though slightly better than that in the series reported by Merrell and Shulman [176], in which 75% of the patients were treated with steroids. An attempt to compare the survivorship in the patients who received a significant degree of steroid therapy with that in patients on a conservative regime was difficult because of the great variation in dosage and duration of treatment. It is interesting that the curves suggest a slightly increased survivorship during the first 18 months in the steroid-treated group, but a slightly decreased survivorship after 5 years (see Fig. 1).

Statistical comparison of the course in patients treated with steroids with that in those not receiving steroids is also hard to interpret. When only patients who received 40 mg/day or more for 2 months or more are considered, there was no correlation with duration of disease, course, or percentage of the patients who died.

Dosage of corticosteroids. The question as to the proper dose of corticosteroids to use in any one patient produces many differences of opinion. As has been discussed, there is no "evidence" on which to base a decision. No statistically sound study has been carried out and perhaps never can be, as stated above, because of the unpredictable exacerbations that could necessitate the breaking of the treatment regimen. Statements abound in the literature supporting the use of specific dose levels without presenting adequate evidence on which to base the recommendations. Difficulty in some of the reports arises from the lack of specific and constant criteria, so that the groups being compared may not all contain patients with the same disease and the variations in severity may not be described. In addition, there is often not adequate knowledge of the course of the disease to allow any interpretation of the effect of therapy. Another frequent defect is a failure to follow the patients for sufficient periods of time. Far too commonly, clinical and especially laboratory improvement, such as a lowered complement level, on a treatment regimen is used as a recommendation for a specific dose or drug, the conclusions as to the value of the recommended therapy not being modified by the fact that the patient or patients on that dose or drug died 2 months later. The conclusions of the report of such a study may refer only to the original improvement and thereupon recommend the treatment, with the result that only critical readers will realize the defect. The greatest differences of opinion arise in relation to the treatment of renal involvement, which will be discussed later.

In the decision as to the dose to use, reliance must again be placed on such empirical evidence as is obtained from relatively large series of patients classified by criteria as specific as possible and followed for several years. Since corticosteroid therapy, with all of the disadvantages discussed above, should be used in as low a dosage as possible for as short a time as feasible, it is wise to start with the lowest dose that empirical experience would indicate may be adequate for the situation. For example, our experience, corroborated by that of others [173], suggests that 40 mg of prednisone a day (10 mg every 6 hours) would be adequate for even moderately severe lupus "crisis" with fever up to 103° or 104°, extreme malaise, headache, often chest pain, rash and joint pains, and moderately severe reduction in levels of hemoglobin (to 6 to 8 gm per 100 ml), platelets (to 40,000 to 60,000 cells per cu mm), and leukocytes (to 2,000 to 3,000 cells per cu mm). In some cases 25 to 30 mg are adequate. With more acute and severe disease, 60 mg of prednisone a day (in four doses) or other steroid, intravenously if necessary, may be advisable. Rarely is a larger dose than the equivalent of 60 mg of prednisone necessary, nor is there evidence that it is of greater effectiveness. Many investigators have recommended higher levels [1, 85, 105, 145, 178, 204], but without adequate evidence. Unfortunately the dramatic situation with such sick patients tends to lead to great pressure, felt by the physician himself and by all concerned, to "do something." Often the "thing" that is done is to increase the dose of steroid even before the effect of the original dose has been determined. Presumably some of the impression that a higher dose is better arises from the fact that the response to the original lower dose may reach its height just after the new dosage is started, the improvement being ascribed incorrectly to the increase in the dose.

The period of time over which the full dose should be continued varies according to the situation in each patient. However, in general, as soon as the majority of the signs and symptoms have shown good response and the patient's condition is adequate, gradual lowering of the dose should be started. In the case of hemolytic anemia, for instance, when the hematocrit has risen from 20% or below to 28%, slow reduction of the dose can be started. In general, it is wise to reduce only by 5 mg when the daily dose is 30 mg or greater, by 2.5 mg when the dose is between 10 or 15 and 30 mg, and by 1 mg when the dose is less than 10 mg a day. Further reduction should not be made while any reaction of any kind to the first withdrawal persists— such as any increased fever, greater malaise, or increased arthralgia. If no reaction has occurred, a second reduction can be made, usually in 3 to 6 days. When a patient has been on steroid therapy for weeks or longer, reduction often can be made only every few weeks or even months.

Of less importance than the dose, probably, is the choice of the individual corticosteroid that is given for treatment. The anti-inflammatory activity varies markedly in terms of activity per mg of drug, but equivalent doses can be approximated. Individual physicians or patients may favor one or another of the effective steroids. The only significant differences probably are slight variations in toxicity. Psychotic disturbances due to steroid therapy were surely more frequent when cortisone was the commonly used corticosteroid. Gastric irritation or even ulceration, common to all, is probably greater with cortisone than with others. Myopathy has been more frequently seen with dexamethasone and triamcinolone.

Treatment of localized areas of rash or resistant skin lesions with ointments containing corticosteroids is sometimes of value. Absorption is limited execpt when large areas are treated.

Intra-articular injection is rarely indicated or necessary in SLE. Joint involvement is occasionally very acute but subsides with treatment of the disease in general. Few troublesome joint symptoms persist as the disease activity decreases. Chronic joint involvement is uncommon, occurring in this series in 30% (43 of 142).

Controversy continues as to any advantage of giving steroid medication every other day, using twice the daily dose. Proponents of this method of therapy argue that equal anti-inflammatory effect may be obtained with fewer of the undesirable side effects of corticosteroid treatment, and that withdrawal of the medication can be carried out with less reaction. Physicians who do not favor every-other-day medication are aware of the lack of any evidence in any studies that the anti-inflammatory effects of steroids can be separated from the other pharmacologic actions of the drugs, including the undesirable side effects. They interpret the decrease in side effects merely as an indication that the total effect of the drug is less as an anti-inflammatory agent also. This is my opinion. Some patients in this series when tried on steroids every second day noted rather marked malaise and fatiguability and occasionally increased joint symptoms during the day without medication, and improvement again after the large dose on the following morning, similar to the findings of Rothfield [212]. In other cases seen since this study, the rate of improvement appeared to increase when medication was changed from every other day to 2 to 3 times a day, a schedule that I prefer. There is, as yet, no evidence by which to solve this problem.

The question as to whether the central nervous system involvement of SLE responds specifically to steroid therapy remains unanswered. Whenever the manifestations appear or increase when steroid therapy is started or the dose is increased, steroids should be withdrawn as rapidly as the activity of the disease permits. Even in patients with central nervous system involvement presumably due entirely to SLE there is no evidence that starting steroid therapy or increasing the dose is of value, though cases with improvement have been reported [69, 221]. In the case of patients with very severe activity of SLE, treatment with corticosteroids is indicated. With improvement of the disease, the nervous system involvement improves as does that of all systems. In my experience in the 64 patients in this series with such involvement there has been improvement in the psychosis or other nervous system involvement attributable specifically to steroid therapy in only 1 patient. In many patients the psychosis has decreased as steroids were withdrawn.

Cytotoxic Drugs

The dysfunction of immunological mechanisms in SLE became more apparent in the period after 1940. Coburn and Moore [49] reported very large amounts of globulin in the plasma of patients with SLE. As a consequence, drugs known to suppress the tissue reaction to immune complexes in animals were tried in the treatment of lupus [64, 68, 89]. The lack of definite alteration in the course of the disease and the marked toxicity of the drugs [250], especially in their effect on hematopoiesis, prevented general acceptance of these drugs in therapy of SLE. More recently the availability of azathioprine and cyclophosphamide and the evidence of their relatively lower immediate toxicity, except in patients in whom they reduce leukocytes too dramatically, have led to increasing use of these drugs in SLE. They are ordinarily not used in the treatment of SLE until corticosteroids have been tried, both because of greater immediate toxicity in many cases and because a widespread therapeutic effect of such drugs compared to corticosteroids has not been demonstrated. Azathioprine has been reported to be effective in treatment of the hemolytic anemia [125, 163]. Evidence is lacking as to its immediate value in severe lupus crisis with high fever, headache, and extensive serositis. Whether any effect of these drugs is determined by their immunosuppressive activity or by a direct anti-inflammatory action has never been established. The lack of correlation between clinical improvement and laboratory evidence of suppression of immune reactions, such as increase in complement levels, suggests that the drugs act, at least in part, directly as anti-inflammatory agents [251].

When patients with severe activity cannot be given corticosteroids or show no improvement after 7 to 10 days of steroid therapy, azathioprine would be given by most physicians and in many cases slow improvement takes place. One encounters the usual difficulty in interpreting how much of the improvement is ascribable to either drug and how much to spontaneous healing. It is seldom necessary to use azathioprine, in my experience, and it should be used with caution. Choice of the dose to be used varies with different investigators. Perhaps the average dose of azathioprine is 3 mg/kg per day in three doses. It is wise to give only 50 mg for 2 to 3 days, then 100 mg for 2 days, and then the full dose. Daily white cell, differential, and platelet counts must be performed for 7 days and then twice a week for 1 month, once a week for 1 month, and then every 2 weeks to 1 month. If a significant reduction in leukocyte count (2,000 to 3,000 cells per cu mm) results, the dose should be lowered and, with continued decrease in leukocyte count, the drug must be omitted. In the case of patients who already have leukopenia when the treatment is started, the deci-

sion as to the reduction in leukocyte count that necessitates a lowering
or omission of the drug is difficult. If a 25% fall in the count occurs,
the dose should be lowered, and with a second decrease in leukocytes
or a fall below 2,000 cells per cu mm, the drug should be omitted. A
significant percentage of patients cannot continue on azathioprine.
Development of malignancy has been reported, as with other cytotoxic drugs [130, 157, 170, 250, 263]. Cyclophosphamide, the other
most commonly used cytotoxic drug in SLE, has also not been proved
to have value in lupus crisis or in any of the system involvements
[251]. The dosage usually given is 2 mg/kg per day in three doses. The
same precautions must be taken in regard to leukopenia as with the
use of azathioprine. One of the other most serious complications is
hemorrhagic cystitis, which may persist after the medication is
stopped. In an attempt to prevent this complication, the 3 daily doses
should be given before 4 P.M. and good fluid intake maintained.

Other cytotoxic drugs, such as 6-mercaptopurine, methotrexate,
nitrogen mustard, and chlorambucil are not commonly employed in
the treatment of SLE. There is no good evidence that they have any
advantage over or any less toxicity than azathioprine or cyclophosphamide.

Antimalarial Drugs

Among the anti-inflammatory drugs often used in the treatment of
SLE are the antimalarials, especially chloroquine and hydroxychloroquine. Without question their most certain value is in treatment of the
skin involvement. While only one statistical study has been carried
out [136], empirical evidence exists as to their value for therapy of the
lupus rash in many patients [69, 97, 103]. They should be prescribed
when skin involvement persists after acute activity of lupus subsides
or where there is chronic skin rash. How much effect these drugs have
on other manifestations of the disease is impossible to state with certainty. An anti-inflammatory effect of chloroquine in rheumatoid
arthritis has been demonstrated by controlled double-blind studies
with random selection of patients [50], but large doses (800 mg) were
used. The general improvement that occurs when some patients with
SLE are given chloroquine or hydroxychloroquine, as in some of this
series, strongly suggests a general anti-inflammatory effect. Many
physicians add these drugs to the therapeutic regime when activity of
the disease is severe or when overall improvement is slow. This is my
practice. Some physicians, however, never use chloroquine or hy-

droxychloroquine because of the danger of irreversible retinal damage. The other toxic manifestations, including gastrointestinal symptoms and deposits in the cornea, may necessitate omission of the drug but they are all reversible. Unfortunately, the damage to the retina often cannot be recognized until it has reached an irreversible stage, though some investigators have detected early changes by measurement of light-induced rise in the corneoretinal potential [43]. It is probably safe to give a dose of 250 mg of chloroquine to patients over the age of 15 or one of 400 mg of hydroxychloroquine for 8 months. In SLE with severe skin involvement responsive to hydroxychloroquine treatment and especially with apparent systemic response, it is occasionally legitimate to continue the medication longer than 8 months, in great contrast to the situation in rheumatoid arthritis in which the relatively mild anti-inflammatory effect does not warrant the risk of treatment prolonged beyond 8 months. In case of crises in SLE or very severe disease, some physicians would prescribe 500 or 750 mg of chloroquine or 800 mg of hydroxychloroquine [69], but doses of this size should not be maintained for more than a few weeks at most.

Treatment of Renal Involvement

In view of the general tendency to consider, probably unwisely, the treatment of the renal involvement of SLE separately from that of other manifestations, the subject will be discussed here in detail. The literature on this aspect of therapy is very extensive and has to be examined critically because of the diverse criteria used in the selection of patients to be included in each series, the relatively small number of patients on which some of the reports are based, and the varied periods of follow-up from which conclusions are drawn. The great difficulty in making any decision regarding the treatment of the renal disease arises from the fact that no controlled double-blind study of any therapy with random selection of patients and adequate follow-up has ever been carried out, and perhaps never can be, as stated above. It is still possible that such a study could be done by a combination of arthritis units with special provision for the patients that would have to be withdrawn. This would be of tremendous value!

Unfortunately, most of the literature is pervaded by an acceptance of the value of corticosteroids in the treatment of renal involvement in SLE, despite the fact that there is no sound evidence of such value. The general belief that corticosteroids are of value and in fact essential in treatment of the renal disease arose for several reasons. Of great importance was the enthusiastic presentation of cases of lupus glomerulonephritis treated with steroids by Pollak et al. [204]. Despite the lack of any controls and the unjustified comparison of the course of the treated patients with that of a group of patients used previously in an excellent histologic study of the features of renal disease in SLE [187], the conclusion that high doses of steroids are not only helpful but essential in the treatment of glomerulonephritis of SLE has been generally accepted and frequently quoted in reports on the treatment of renal disease in lupus [1, 178, 243]. Even subsequent clinical studies indicating that the overall course in lupus patients with renal disease probably is not better with high (60 mg or more) doses of prednisone than with lower doses (20 to 30 mg or less) [59, 109, 173, 214] have not prevented frequent references to the necessity for high doses. Another extremely important reason for the general belief in the value of steroids in the treatment of the renal involvement of SLE is the marked improvement in renal function and urinary findings that usually accompanies improvement in other manifestations of the disease when steroids are used in the treatment of lupus crisis or severe activity of the disease. Unfortunately, little known and never quoted is the similar improvement in renal manifestations that takes place when severe activity of the disease subsides under any treatment such as aspirin or immunosuppressive drugs or spontaneously (see Appendix, cases 1, 3, 4, 12). A similar observation was made by Baldwin et al. [18] in the case of focal nephritis. Obviously the marked improvement as lupus crisis is controlled gives no indication that corticosteroid therapy alters the long-term course of renal disease in SLE and no evidence on which to base the premise that steroid therapy should always be used in the treatment of diffuse renal involvement, as suggested by others [60, 69]. The relatively poorer prognostic significance of diffuse as compared to focal glomerular changes in SLE is well supported by studies by several investigators [18, 47, 53, 187], but none of their findings proves the value of prolonged steroid therapy in diffuse involvement.

The other drugs suggested by many for prolonged treatment of renal disease in SLE are the so-called cytotoxic drugs. The rationale for their use is the known effect of these drugs in the inflammation produced by immune complexes in animals, and the demonstration of the components of such complexes, as DNA, γ globulin, and complement, in the glomeruli in the renal disease of lupus. However, as discussed above, the evidence of immunosuppression, such as raising of complement levels in the blood, does not always correlate with any indication of clinical improvement. This lack of correlation suggests that the drugs act, at least in part, as anti-inflammatory agents. The drugs that have been tried are 6-mercaptopurine, methotrexate, nitrogen mustard, chlorambucil, cyclophosphamide, and azathioprine. The reports of their use suffer from all of the difficulties discussed above and there is no sound evidence for the value of any of them in the renal involvement of SLE except for improvement in renal disease which is part of a general response to treatment in severe active disease. This gives no evidence for their subsequent value in affecting the course of the renal involvement. The relatively lesser toxicity of azathioprine and the suggestive empirical evidence of improvement in renal disease with long-term treatment has led to relatively greater use of this drug. However, its toxicity, including the possible development of malignancy [130, 157, 170, 250], has raised the question of the advisability of such treatment.

Reported series treated with azathioprine or cyclophosphamide are small and uncontrolled or have short follow-up periods [2, 66, 163, 178, 251, 259]. Since the evidence of the present series and other reports indicates that slow improvement from severe renal disease to normal function and urinary findings can take place without the use of azathioprine, cyclophosphamide, or corticosteroids (see Appendix, case 1), and since the number of cases that improved similarly on the cytotoxic drugs, as reported in the literature, is small, there is little reason to argue that patients with severe or worsening renal disease must be treated with azathioprine or cyclophosphamide (or with corticosteroids, as already discussed). Exacerbation of lupus after withdrawal of azathioprine has been reported [231, 259] and has been seen by us in a few cases.

The present series cannot properly be used in direct comparison with the groups in which the results of renal biopsies have been used to classify patients into groups. In this series, the dangers of renal biopsy have, in general, been thought to outweigh the slight improvement in classification of patients and to be warranted routinely only if adequately controlled, blindfold studies were being carried out. However, some patients in this series treated with the conservative regimen using aspirin as the anti-inflammatory agent surely had severe, diffuse glomerular involvement with findings such as creatinine clearances of

20 to 30 ml in 24 hours, BUN levels of 100 mg per 100 ml, urinary findings of 10-15 gm of albumin per 24 hours, and 20 to 200 red cells with cellular casts (as in cases 1 and 2). The final return of renal function to normal or near normal levels and duration of life for many years are comparable to the best results reported with other drugs. Zweiman et al. [287] were impressed with the variations in the course of lupus nephritis from patient to patient. Once again arises the difficulty in estimating what percentage of patients would improve on any regimen and maintain good renal function. Estimation of prognosis in any one patient on any regimen remains impossible, despite the fact that individual findings such as a mild or severe degree of renal involvement offer some indication of prognosis. Disturbing, however, are the few patients who have very mild or no clinically evident renal involvement at first but develop severe progressive glomerulonephritis and die in a few years (see Appendix, case 17).

Our experience with dialysis for renal failure in SLE has been very limited. One patient had a severe generalized exacerbation of lupus after she had had relatively mild disease with only a little evidence of renal involvement for years. During the exacerbation renal failure progressed rapidly to a BUN of 170 mg and a creatinine of 4 mg per 100 ml. With peritoneal dialysis there was little control of the serum levels of urea nitrogen and creatinine and severe lupus activity persisted. Death occurred 4 days after dialysis was started. A more fortunate result has occurred in a patient with severe residual renal failure (BUN 232 mg and creatinine 12 mg per 100 ml) but relatively inactive lupus. Hemodialysis three times a week has produced good control of the levels after dialysis of BUN (20 mg) and creatinine (5.2 mg), the patient's general condition has improved, the disease has remained relatively inactive, and the patient has been able to carry on many normal activities. Kidney transplants have not been performed in our series.

Summary

In summary, the treatment of the renal involvement in SLE remains an integral part of the treatment of the disease as a whole, and should not, in itself, require any specific program. In all patients with lupus an attempt to produce remission should be made. In many patients this can be accomplished with the basic conservative regimen described above with the use of only aspirin or aspirin and hydroxy-chloroquine as the anti-inflammatory agents. With greater severity of disease, as in lupus crisis, with or without severe renal disease, other anti-inflammatory drugs such as corticosteroids or azathioprine or cyclophosphamide may be necessary. Unfortunately, many reported series suffer from various difficulties, so it is impossible even to estimate what percentage of patients with renal disease would improve markedly and live for many years on any one regimen, or to be dogmatic as to which drug is best.

One need no longer approach a patient with the gloom of a 65% mortality in less than 5 years, but rather with the optimism of 60% or more survivorship for 15 years or more. This difference in a physician's belief is readily transmitted to the patient. Many a member of the house staff or visiting staff has said to me, "Oh, the patient doesn't know that I feel discouraged." This I do not believe. The feeling is transmitted in many ways, especially if an able physician has a good relationship with his patient, and it may be very detrimental. It surely does not add to the emotional relaxation which many of us consider an essential part of the treatment of this disease. If such discouragement (with focus on 80% mortality in a few years) were entirely justified, one could only hope to conceal it from the patient, but in the present situation of perhaps only 35 to 40% mortality in many years, one can actively encourage.

Appendix: Case Reports

Cases 1 through 4 demonstrate the improvement in the renal involvement when the activity of the disease subsides. Case 1 was treated with aspirin, cases 2 and 3 with steroids also, as indicated on the figures, and case 4 with prednisone, hydroxychloroquine, nitrogen mustard, and cyclophosphamide, at various times.

Case 1 (Fig. A 1). This 43-year-old white woman was admitted to the Massachusetts General Hospital in November 1954 with a complaint of upper abdominal pain. Two years before admission she had had pain in joints with an upper respiratory infection. A similar episode occurred 4 months before admission and 4 weeks later she noted fatigue, slight fever, joint pains, pain in the right flank and epigastrium, a nonproductive cough, slight swelling around her eyes, and abdominal swelling. Symptoms increased slowly. Three weeks before admission a chest x-ray was reported to show a large pleural effusion on the right. Examination on admission showed a temperature of 101° rectally which rose to 104° on the third day; pulse 120, respiration 30; blood pressure (BP) 95/65; puffy eyelids, generalized lymphadenopathy, dullness and decreased breath sounds at right base, liver palpable 3 cm below costal margin. Laboratory findings showed urine with 2+ albumin, many white cells, and a few hyaline and granular casts; hemoglobin 8.6 gm per 100 ml; leukocyte count 5,650 with 75% neutrophils; NPN 14 mg per 100 ml, serum albumin 2.8 gm per 100 ml, and globulin 2.6 gm. Chest x-ray showed right pleural effusion; electrocardiogram showed low voltage and inverted T waves. Urine cultures were negative. She remained very sick for 4 weeks. Fever fluctuated from 100° to 104° R, cytoid bodies appeared in the fundi, mouth lesions developed and a macular rash appeared on arms and back. After 1 month gradual improvement occurred with lessening of pleural fluid and ascites, and with decrease in fever and weakness. She was treated with 4.5

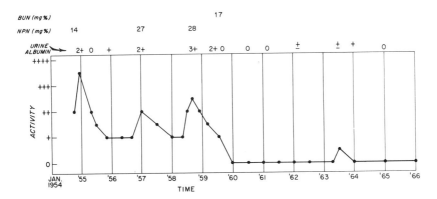

Figure A1. Course of systemic lupus erythematosus from onset in case 1. The symbols 0, +, ++, +++, and ++++ indicate arbitrary estimates of the total activity of the disease. This patient was treated conservatively.

gm of aspirin daily and bed rest. After 3 months she was discharged for convalescence to another hospital and remained there 3 months. When seen here
at that time she was free of symptoms except for moderate fatiguability.
Examination was normal. Urine was normal; hematocrit 40% and leukocyte
count 4,600. She remained well, leading a fairly normal life for 6 months.
However, in September 1956 she was readmitted because of a breast mass. A
radical mastectomy showed an adenocarcinoma with metastases in 9 of 31
lymph nodes. Following the operation she had fatiguability and joint pains
which persisted for 1 year. Then she felt well again for 10 months, when she
had an upper respiratory infection followed by extreme fatigue, anorexia, and
intermittent fever to 102°. She was readmitted in September 1958. Examination showed temperature 102°, pulse 130, BP 100/65, a mottled rash over
neck and shoulders; liver palpable 4 cm below costal margin; spleen tip palpable. Laboratory findings were: urine with 2 to 3 + albumin, 10-20 red cells
per high-power field, many granular casts and a few red cell casts; hematocrit
27%; leukocyte count 3,750 per high-power field with 80% neutrophils; many
LE cells; NPN 28 mg per 100 ml; creatinine clearance was 38 liters per 24
hours; and serum albumin was 2.5 gm per 100 ml and globulin 4.0 gm. EKG
was normal. On a regimen of bed rest, aspirin, and transfusion she improved
steadily and was discharged on the same regimen in 3 weeks. In 6 months she
had become entirely free of symptoms on her normal activities and urine was
free of albumin. She remained well except for slight fatiguability in 1963 during the depression following her husband's death.

Since the series closed there has been no exacerbation of lupus but she developed a mass in the other breast in 1970 with widespread metastases. These
have responded fairly well to treatment.

This case demonstrates the marked improvement and finally complete
remission of the disease on a regimen of bed rest and full doses of aspirin.

Case 2 (Fig. A 2). This 27-year-old white man was admitted in May 1942 with
a complaint of joint pain and swelling of 18 months' duration. For 6 months
he had had a rash over cheeks and nose. He had lost 20 pounds during the past
year. Urine examination 2 months before admission showed 2 + albumin.
Examination on admission showed an erythematous maculopapular rash in
butterfly distribution. Joints showed marked swelling of all of the proximal
phalangeal joints. Spleen was palpable 2 cm below the costal margin and there
was generalized lymphadenopathy. Laboratory examination showed 2 +
albumin and occasional red and white cells and hyaline casts. Hemoglobin
was 16 gm per 100 ml and leukocyte count 5,000 with 50% neutrophils. Sedimentation rate 0.72 mm per min. Serum albumin was 4.9 gm per 100 ml and
globulin 2.9 gm. On a regimen of bed rest and aspirin he improved and was
discharged in 3 weeks. When seen 2 months later he felt quite well except for
occasional stiffness of joints and intermittent recurrence of the rash. He continued on bed rest and aspirin but 2 months later returned to work and noted
increased fatiguability and joint pains. Examination and laboratory findings
remained the same. He increased his periods of rest. His condition remained
good for 1 year, at which time his rash became worse and some swelling of

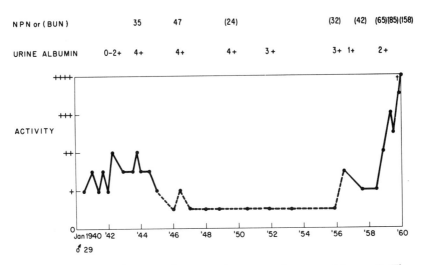

| N P N or (B U N) | | 35 | 47 | (24) | | | (32) | (42) | (65)(85)(158) |
| URINE ALBUMIN | 0-2+ | 4+ | 4+ | 4+ | 3+ | | 3+ | 1+ | 2+ |

Figure A2. Course of systemic lupus erythematosus from onset in case 2. The symbols 0, +, + +, + + +, and + + + + indicate arbitrary estimates of the total activity of the disease. This patient was treated conservatively.

ankles appeared following hard work and exposure to sun. Examination showed increase in the rash on face and behind ears, and pitting edema. One month later the edema involved entire legs and scrotum. There was generalized lymphadenopathy; spleen was palpable 4 cm below the costal margin and liver 3 cm. Urine showed 4 + albumin, sedimentation rate was 1.7 mm/min, hematocrit was 38%, serum albumin was 1.7 gm per 100 ml and globulin 1.8 gm. He continued to work but spent the rest of the time in bed and continued aspirin. The edema subsided slowly over the next 2 months, and the rash improved. Urine continued to show 4 + albumin and had 30-60 red cells and 15-20 white cells per high-power field for 6 months, when the cells decreased to normal. The hematocrit fell to 32%. NPN rose to 44 mg per 100 ml. His general condition improved and he was very well for 12 years. He worked full time and went to night school. When seen in 1956 examination was normal except for BP 160/110. Urine showed + albumin. BUN was 29 mg per 100 ml. In the following three years he had occasional anginal pain and blood pressure rose gradually to 190/110. He developed dyspnea, nausea, and vomiting and was admitted to another hospital. BUN was 85 mg per 100 ml. He improved symptomatically with hemodialysis and was able to return to work for 2 months. Nausea and vomiting recurred and he was readmitted to the same hospital. BUN was 152 mg per 100 ml and creatinine 19.8 mg. Hemodialysis was of no benefit and he died one month later. Postmortem examination showed severe glomerulonephritis with much proliferation, many adhesions, many glomeruli hyalinized; acute and chronic pericarditis, acute pleuritis, focal myocarditis and mild healed valvulitis.

This patient had an excellent remission of the activity of the disease for over 10 years, despite some persistent reduction of renal function.

Case 3 (Fig. A 3). This 17-year-old white woman was first seen in August 1962, with no complaints except slight fatiguability. She had been well until 5 years before this visit when she had had fever and myalgia. Hemoglobin at that time was 7.8 gm per 100 ml; leukocyte count was 4,300 per cu mm; platelet count was 84,000; LE cells were not seen; and serologic test for syphilis was reported as "false positive." She responded well to treatment with 40 mg of prednisone and the dose was lowered steadily to zero in 2 months. She was free of symptoms except for occasional arthralgia for 5 months. However, hemoglobin decreased again and she was given methylprednisolone (Medrol) 4 mg b.i.d. She continued on this regimen and when seen by another physician in September 1958 she was free of symptoms. Hemoglobin was 10.1 gm per 100 ml, and urine was normal. LE cells were seen. She continued to be free of symptoms for 5 months, when arthralgias developed and she was given aspirin with relief. Five months later she developed a rash over her nose following exposure to intensive sunlight. Fatigue occurred 2 months later, hemoglobin was 9 gm per 100 ml, and the methylprednisolone dose was increased to 12 mg a day. Two months later effusions were noted in both knees. Because of visible side effects of steroid therapy, the dose of methylprednisolone was reduced slowly to 2 mg a day and chloroquine, 250 mg per day, was started. She improved steadily and was free of symptoms in 4 months. Methylprednisolone was discontinued. Hemoglobin and white count were normal and no LE cells were seen but antinuclear antibodies were present. Three months later chloroquine was discontinued. She remained free of all symptoms for 7 months, when joint pain recurred. Chloroquine was restarted. She was again free of symptoms in the 4 months before her first visit to M.G.H. Examination

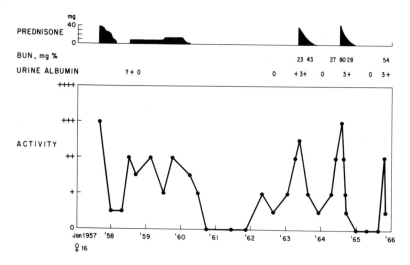

Figure A3. Course of systemic lupus erythematosus from onset in case 3. The symbols 0, +, ++, +++, and ++++ indicate arbitrary estimates of the total activity of the disease. This patient received steroids as indicated.

at that time was normal. Blood pressure was 120/80. Urine was negative except that it was loaded with white cells. Culture was negative. Hemoglobin was 12.1 gm per 100 ml, leukocyte count 6,000. She continued to be free of symptoms for 7 months, when she gained weight rapidly and noted swelling of her ankles, fatiguability, and slight fever. She was admitted to the hospital in April 1963. Examination remained negative except for some edema of legs. Urine showed + albuminuria which increased to 3 +; hemoglobin was 8.4 gm per 100 ml; serum albumin was 2.6 gm per 100 ml and globulin 2.3 gm; cholesterol 227 mg per 100 ml, and creatinine 1.1 mg; creatinine clearance was 48 liters in 24 hours. Sedimentation rate was 0.75 mm per min. Because of the hemolytic anemia she was given 42 mg of prednisone a day. The dose was gradually reduced to zero over 5 months. During this period she became free of symptoms. In December 1963, urine was free of albumin and creatinine clearance was 146 liters in 24 hours. Sedimentation rate was 0.52 mm per min. She was working full time. Four months later she had slight swelling of ankles and urine showed 3 + albumin. Hematocrit was 28. She was readmitted in May 1964. Because of a drop in hemoglobin to 7.3 gm per 100 ml, she was started on prednisone, 40 mg a day. The dose was reduced quickly to 20 mg and then slowly to zero over 6 months. She became symptom-free and returned to work in September 1964. Seven months later urine had become free of albumin again, hematocrit was 38 and sedimentation rate was 0.25 mm per min. She again remained well until September 1965, when marked fatiguability recurred and she noted slight swelling of feet and face. Weight increased 8 pounds. She was admitted to another hospital in October 1965. Urine showed albumin, and a hematocrit of 30%. On bed rest and aspirin, her hematocrit rose to 39% and weight fell 4 pounds. However, 1 month later she had an upper respiratory infection and noted increased fatiguability and slight arthralgia. On readmission to the M.G.H. examination was normal, except for some ecchymoses on the lower legs and slight periorbital edema. Serum creatinine was 1.2 mg per 100 ml.

After the series closed, she remained in the hospital because of increasing edema and a fall in platelet count to 50,000 per cu mm. She was treated with 40 mg of prednisone and platelet count rose dramatically, but edema increased and BUN rose to 90 mg/100 ml and creatinine 1.8 mg with a clearance of 30 liters in 24 hours. Two months later there was gradual improvement. She continued to have episodes of nephrosis and increasing renal failure. Hemodialysis 3 times a week has been carried out for the past 4 years. She has done very well, carrying on some normal activities. There has been little evidence of activity of lupus.

The remissions in this patient were accompanied by dramatic decrease in BUN and improvement in creatinine clearance.

Case 4 (Fig. A 4). This 16-year-old white woman was admitted in April 1961. Three years before admission she had a urinary tract infection which apparently cleared completely on treatment. Three months before admission she noted fatiguability, pain and slight swelling of proximal interphalangeal joints and ankles, and facial rash. Hemoglobin was 8 gm per 100 ml. Examination

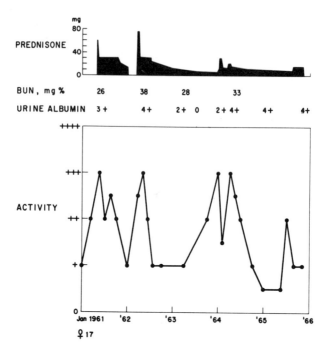

Figure A4. Course of systemic lupus erythematosus from onset in case 4. The symbols 0, +, + +, + + +, and + + + + indicate arbitrary estimates of the total activity of the disease. This patient received steroids as indicated.

on admission showed a temperature of 101° rectally, pulse 80, BP 120/80, a reddish-purple rash in butterfly distribution; lymphadenopathy in posterior, cervical, and axillary areas; spleen palpable 2 cm below the costal margin; and fusiform swelling of the proximal interphalangeal joints. Laboratory findings were: 3+ albuminurea with 40-50 red cells, 8-10 leukocytes per high-power field, and many casts including red-cell casts; hemoglobin 10 gm per 100 ml; leukocyte count 5,000 with 51% neutrophils; BUN 26 mg per 100 ml, and creatinine 1.4 mg with a clearance of 50 liters per day; and many LE cells. Serum albumin was 2.9 gm per 100 ml and globulin 3.5 gm with a slight increase in γ globulin. Chest x-ray was negative. On a regimen of prednisone (60 mg reduced to 45 mg after 1 day) and aspirin, she improved rapidly symptomatically. BUN fell to 18 mg per 100 ml but urinary findings were unchanged. She was discharged after 5 weeks on bed rest, prednisone 30 mg and aspirin 4 gm a day. Following discharge, she remained free of symptoms, with the exception of fatiguability and slight swelling of face and ankles.

She was readmitted in June because of anemia with a hemoglobin of 7 gm per 100 ml. Examination showed temperature 99°, BP 140/84; and slight rash on cheeks and around base of neck. Liver was palpable 3 cm below costal margin. There was 2+ edema of ankles. Urinalysis showed 2+ albumin and 20-25 red cells with rare white-cell casts. BUN was 22 mg per 100 ml and creatinine 0.9 mg. Serum albumin was 2.3 gm per 100 ml and globulin 2.3 gm. Serum cholesterol was 300 mg per 100 ml. She received three transfusions of packed cells; and hemoglobin rose to 14.7 gm per 100 ml. On the sixth day, she was discharged on 25 mg of prednisone and 4.0 gm of aspirin. She remained entirely free of symptoms for 4 months, when she had "dizziness" for 4 days. Laboratory examinations at that time were unchanged except that creatinine clearance was 71 liters per day with a serum creatinine of 1.1 mg per 100 ml. She continued on the same regimen with slow reduction of her prednisone dose to 12.5 mg per day, and remained symptom-free and returned to school in early 1962. Six weeks later swelling of eyes and ankles developed and she gained 10 pounds in weight. On readmission, examination showed BP 134/82 and persistence of Cushingoid features; liver and spleen unchanged; 3 to 4 + edema of ankles and lower legs. Urinary findings were unchanged; hemoglobin 11.5 gm per 100 ml; BUN 38 mg per 100 ml; creatinine clearance 114 liters per day with serum creatinine of 1.0 mg per 100 ml; serum albumin of 1.9 gm per 100 ml and globulin of 2.4 gm. On a regimen of 80 mg of prednisone and diuretics, and subsequently 600 mg of hydroxychloroquine, there was gradual loss of weight to normal over 2 months. She was again free of symptoms and did very well for 16 months. She continued to take 12.5 mg of prednisone daily. Urine albumin decreased to +; granular casts persisted.

Suddenly she developed an upper respiratory infection and 2 days later, in December 1963, was readmitted with a temperature of 106°, pulse 120 and BP 70/30. Examination and chest x-ray showed right lower lobe pneumonia. Hemoglobin was 12.1 gm per 100 ml and leukocyte count 13,900 per cu mm with 74% neutrophils. Urine showed 3 + albumin, 3-4 red cells, 20-30 white cells and 5-6 granular casts per high-power field. BUN was 28 mg per 100 ml; creatinine 2.2 mg per 100 ml; albumin was 2.4 gm and globulin 2.4 gm per 100 ml. LE cells were seen. On a regimen of mannitol intravenously, penicillin, and 200 mg of hydrocortisone intravenously over two days, followed by prednisone 15 mg t.i.d., she improved steadily and was discharged in 2 weeks on prednisone 10 mg b.i.d. Creatinine had fallen to 0.6 mg per 100 ml with a clearance of 142 liters per day. Following discharge, she felt quite well but urine albumin, which had fallen to zero, increased to 4 + and increasing edema appeared 2 months later. She was readmitted in March 1964. Examination showed Cushingoid features, temperature 98.6°, BP 138/100, and spleen palpable 2 cm and liver 3 cm below costal margin. There was 3 + pitting edema of feet and ankles. Urine showed 4 + albumin, 100 red cells and 200 white cells, and 3-5 granular casts per high-power field, and occasional red- and white-cell casts. Hematocrit was 37% and leukocyte count 4,500 per cu mm with 79% neutrophils. BUN was 33 mg and creatinine 1.0 mg per 100 ml. Clearance was 104 liters in 24 hours. She was treated with continued prednisone of 5 mg t.i.d., spironolactone (Aldactone), and hydroxychloroquine 200 mg b.i.d. She began to lose weight in 1 week and was discharged in 2 weeks. For the next 2 years she did quite well on fairly normal activities with no symptoms except for a 1-month episode in 1965 of ankle swelling, treated with increased dose of chlorothiazide and spironolactone.

After the series had ended, she was readmitted in November 1966, and again in March 1967; October 1967; January 1968; December 1970; and finally in January 1971. Creatinine had risen to 2.6 mg per 100 ml in March 1967, and 5.8 mg in January 1968, and 5.2 mg in January 1971, with a BUN of 115 mg per 100 ml. She remained on prednisone, 10 to 30 mg, and on aspirin. Nitrogen mustard was given in November 1967, and cyclophosphamide in December 1970. She died in 1971. Postmortem examination showed a perforation of a diverticulum of the sigmoid colon and hemorrhagic pneumonia. The kidneys showed extensive interstitial fibrosis and hyalinization of many glomeruli. Some glomeruli showed "wire-loop" lesions.

Improvement in this case occurred each time with hospitalization and a variety of drugs in addition to prednisone.

Cases 5 and 6 manifested a mild type of disease with no severe exacerbations. Conservative therapy with aspirin as the only anti-inflammatory agent was given to case 5, low doses of prednisone to case 6.

Case 5 (Fig. A 5). This 15-year-old white female was first seen in 1935 in the outpatient clinic with a complaint of a rash on her face which had developed after she had been in the sun frequently for weeks. Past history was negative. Examination showed a rash in butterfly distribution. She was treated with

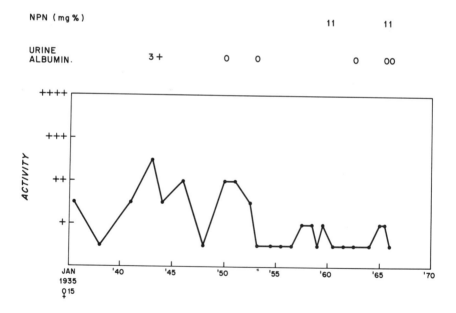

Figure A5. Course of systemic lupus erythematosus from onset in case 5. The symbols +, ++, +++, and ++++ indicate arbitrary estimates of the total activity of the disease. This patient was treated conservatively.

gold. The facial rash disappeared in 4 to 5 months but skin lesions developed on arms and in scalp. The facial rash reappeared in 1941 and was present intermittently until 1943, when she became pregnant. The skin cleared during pregnancy but she had fever and pain in the right costovertebral angle. For 1 year after delivery she was weak and dizzy. One and one-half years after delivery skin lesions reappeared on face, arms, and back, and disappeared and recurred intermittently. In June 1950 she noted pains in hands, elbows, and left thigh. Painful nodules appeared over wrists and metacarpalphalangeal joints. Examination showed temperature 98.6°, BP 128/94; a maculopapular eruption on face and arms. Wrists were swollen and warm. Laboratory examination showed urine normal, hemoglobin 13.4 gm, leukocyte count 5,800 per cu mm, with 56% neutrophils. Sedimentation rate was 0.73 mm/min. No LE cells were seen; BUN was 11 mg/100 ml. For the subsequent 15 years she continued to have a scaly blotchy rash on face and upper back; some fatiguability; occasional joint pains. In 1959 laboratory examination showed a leukocyte count of 4,400 per cu mm. Sedimentation rate remained elevated. LE cells were never seen. In 1965 she was admitted to the hospital because of attacks of chest pain. There was some relief from nitroglycerine. On examination heart was negative; blood pressure 170/100. Laboratory examination showed hematocrit of 33%, reticulocyte count of 15%, and platelet count of 44,000 per cu mm. Electrocardiogram showed transient T-wave abnormalities. Serial enzyme determinations were normal. A diagnosis of coronary artery disease was made and the possibility that it was due to lupus was discussed. Following discharge she felt well on a regimen of pentaerythritol tetranitrate and buffered aspirin.

She has continued to do well. This patient had only mild disease for approximately 20 years and then almost full remission for 10 years. She was treated with a conservative regimen.

Case 6 (Fig. A 6). This 39-year-old white woman was admitted in 1956 with the complaint of intermittent swelling, redness, stiffness, and pain of hands and wrists of 1 year's duration. Six months before admission there was sudden onset of severe abdominal pain and nausea, treated with sulfonamides. Four days later a rash appeared on her nose and eyebrows. Five months later, after a period of overwork, the rash spread to the cheeks and became much redder. Past history revealed repeated false-positive serologic tests for 12 years; an attack of virus pneumonia lasting 4 to 6 weeks, 6 years before admission; an atypical sunburn 3 years before admission, which left residual pigmentation over the malar eminences; and "anemia" noted 1 year before admission. Physical examination revealed temperature 98.8°, BP 120/70; a very anxious patient, an erythematous eruption with slight plugging over butterfly area and in eyebrows; slightly enlarged firm lymph nodes in cervical, axillary, and inguinal areas; liver dullness 2 cm below the costal margin. Laboratory examination showed trace to 2+ albuminuria; numerous granular and hyaline casts; white cell count of 5,000 per cu mm with 44% neutrophils; hemoglobin of 14 gm/100 ml; sedimentation rate of 40 mm/hr. LE cells were found in the blood. Electrocardiogram was normal except for minor ST changes. X-rays of

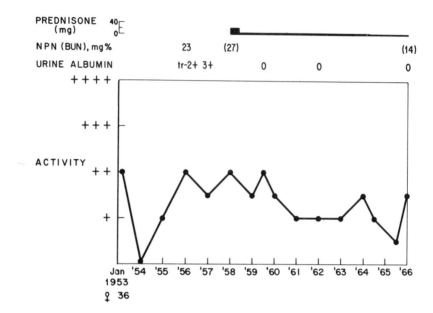

Figure A6. Course of systemic lupus erythematosus from onset in case 6. The symbols +, ++, +++, and ++++ indicate arbitrary estimates of the total activity of the disease. This patient was treated with steroids as indicated.

chest and abdomen were normal. Biopsy of skin on the cheek was consistent with lupus erythematosus. Hinton test was positive. NPN was 23 mg/100 ml. Electrophoretic pattern of serum proteins showed increased γ globulins.

For 10 years after discharge she was followed at various hospitals and in general did very well. However, because of an increase in symptoms she was started on prednisone, 20 mg a day in 1958, reduced to 5 mg in a few months. When seen here in 1966, she had continued to work full time as a secretary. She had had intermittent joint pain and swelling, fatiguability had increased, and she had noted some shortness of breath when climbing stairs. The steroid dosage had been reduced to 2.5 mg per day. General examination in 1966 was normal except for some swelling of the metacarpophalangeal and proximal interphalangeal joints. Laboratory examinations showed normal urine; hemoglobin, 7.8 gm per 100 ml; leukocyte count, 4,050 cells per cu mm; reticulocyte count, 1.6%; serum creatinine, 0.8 mg/100 ml; sedimentation rate, 36 mm/hour; and serum iron, 35 μgm per 100 ml. Serum electrophoresis showed increased γ globulins; electrocardiogram was normal; LE cell test was negative; and urine urobilinogen was 1.1 Ehrlich units.

When last seen in 1970, she had continued to do well.

Despite the fact that this patient had mild disease only, she had been treated with prednisone.

Cases 7 and 8 demonstrate the severe, steadily downhill type of course. Case 7 received aspirin only, case 8 prednisone in high doses.

Case 7 (Fig. A 7). This 33-year-old white man, a machine shop worker, was admitted in 1946 with the complaint of swelling of the face for 5 months and joint pains and swelling for 3 months. One week before admission he noted weakness and fever. During the illness he had lost 20 pounds. Past history was noncontributory. Physical examination revealed temperature 101° rectally; blood pressure 130/90; pulse 100; marked periorbital edema with a violaceous color; pigmentation over forehead and at base of nails; generalized lymphadenopathy; splenomegaly; tenderness, swelling, and pain on motion in proximal phalangeal and metacarpophalangeal joints, wrists, elbows, knees, and ankles. Laboratory examination showed 0 to 2+ albuminuria, no red blood cells or casts; leukocyte count of 3,500 per cu mm, with 58% neutrophils; hemoglobin of 11.3 gm per 100 ml; and sedimentation rate of 1.4 mm per min (normal up to 0.35 mm). NPN was 26 mg per 100 ml. Electrocardiogram showed low voltage QRS and flat T_1 and T_{CF45} and low T waves in the other leads. Chest x-ray was normal. X-rays of hands showed some decalcification of the ends of the bones.

Course: On a regimen of bed rest and aspirin, he improved considerably and was discharged after 7 weeks. However, he soon had recurrence of swelling of

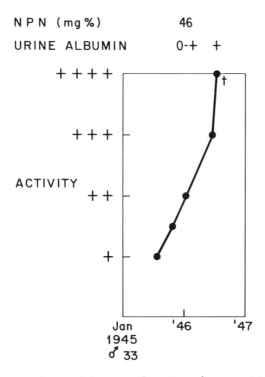

Figure A7. Course of systemic lupus erythematosus from onset in case 7. The symbols +, ++, +++, and ++++ indicate arbitrary estimates of the total activity of the disease. This patient was treated conservatively.

his eyes and increased fatigue. Two months later he was admitted to another hospital. Examination was essentially the same as on the previous admission. His condition deteriorated and he died 1 month later.

This case represents severe, rapidly fatal disease without renal involvement.

Case 8 (Fig. A 8). This 36-year-old black woman was first seen in the outpatient clinic in January 1962 with a complaint of diffuse joint pains of 2 months' duration. She had been well until 3 months before this visit, when she noted weakness. For 1 month she had had nausea and vomiting. Past history

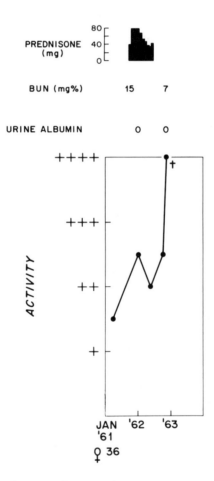

Figure A8. Course of systemic lupus erythematosus from onset in case 8. The symbols +, ++, +++, and ++++ indicate arbitrary estimates of the total activity of the disease. This patient was treated with steroids as indicated.

was negative except for an attack of "acute rheumatic fever" at the age of 12 when she was in the West Indies. Physical examination was negative except for pain on motion of fingers, wrists, shoulders, neck, and lower back, and slight anterior cervical and axillary lymphadenopathy. BP was 110/65, pulse 81. Laboratory examination showed urine analysis negative; leukocyte count 3,500 per cu mm with 42% neutrophils; hemoglobin 8.9 gm per 100 ml; sedimentation rate 3 mm per hr; Hinton test positive; treponema pallidum immobilization test negative. Many LE cells were seen; latex fixation test for rheumatoid factor was 1:160; chest x-rays showed slight enlargement of the heart, and slight prominence of the hilar regions. She improved slightly on rest and aspirin, but 6 weeks later she developed left anterior chest pain. She had lost 30 pounds and had begun to have night sweats. She was admitted to the hospital. Physical examination was unchanged except for generalized lymphadenopathy; splenomegaly and hepatomegaly (both 3 cm below the costal margin); and decrease in joint pain. Laboratory examination showed urine negative; leukocyte count 12,800 with 58% neutrophils, hematocrit 26% with 19% reticulocyte. Urine urobilinogen was 18 Ehrlich units. Chest x-ray showed slight generalized enlargement of the heart as before. Electrocardiogram was within normal limits. Hilar areas appeared normal. Serum albumin was 3.4 gm per 100 ml and globulin 6.4 gm. Serum electrophoresis showed a marked increase in the γ-globulin fraction. An axillary lymph node biopsy showed lymphoid hyperplasia. Bone marrow revealed erythroid hyperplasia.

Course: She was given 10 mg of prednisone 4 times a day for 12 days, with clinical improvement. However, because of minimal rise of the hemoglobin, the dose of prednisone was increased to 20 mg 4 times a day. Clinical and laboratory improvement continued and she was discharged on the same dose of prednisone after 10 days. One week later she developed polyuria, polydypsia, and glycosuria requiring treatment with orinase. She developed a perianal abscess and was readmitted in June. Physical examination was the same as that in February except for acneiform lesions on face; decreased adenopathy; no splenomegaly or hepatomegaly; and a perianal abscess 2 cm in diameter. Laboratory examination showed urine normal; hematocrit 40%, leukocyte count 7,800 with 80% neutrophils. Serum albumin was 3.8 gm per 100 ml; and serum globulin 3.5 gm. Chest x-ray was unchanged. Following drainage of the abscess she was discharged. Slow improvement continued but 1 month later, 4 days after her last visit to the outpatient clinic, she died suddenly. Postmortem examination disclosed a confluent bronchopneumonia of the posterior lobes and focal thickening of the basement membrane of the glomeruli.

Very severe disease in this patient was not controlled on a regimen of bed rest, aspirin, and prednisone. Severe, terminal pneumonitis is seen frequently in patients with SLE, especially when they are receiving steroids.

Cases 9 and 10 illustrate the severe, downhill type of course with only short remissions. Case 9 was treated with a conservative regimen, case 10 with steroids in moderate doses.

Case 9 (Fig. A9). This 23-year-old white woman was admitted in 1941 because of joint and chest pain. Three years before admission, she developed generalized joint pains. Eight months later, a rash appeared on her cheeks (following sun exposure) and she became very sick with high fever. She had patchy alopecia. After 4 months in another hospital, rash and joint pains disappeared and she returned to work. In 6 months, the joint pains and swelling and facial rash recurred. Again she was very sick with temperature of 107°, delirium, total alopecia, and oral ulcerations. Symptoms and signs subsided after 2 months in another hospital except for the persistence of some facial rash. She became pregnant soon thereafter and had no symptoms during pregnancy except for pleuritic pain for 5 weeks in the fourth and fifth months. Sixteen days before admission she delivered a normal baby. The pleuritic pain returned following delivery, and she developed joint pain and swelling, sore

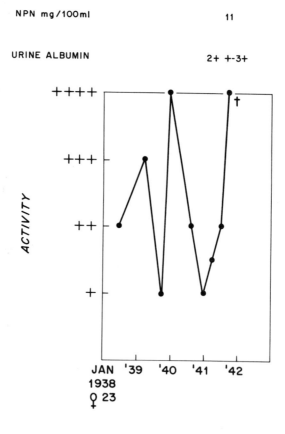

Figure A9. Course of systemic lupus erythematosus from onset in case 9. The symbols +, ++, +++, and ++++ indicate arbitrary estimates of the total activity of the disease. This patient was treated conservatively.

mouth, alopecia, and fever of 104°. She had profuse lochial discharge from which nonhemolytic streptococcus was grown. Physical examination showed respiratory difficulty with severe anterior chest pains on breathing. Temperature was 102°, BP 110/70, there was an erythematous rash over the cheeks and nose with some areas of atrophy. All joints were painful and right knee was swollen. Chest showed slight dullness at left base. Laboratory examination showed 3 + albuminuria, many white cells in the urine; hemoglobin 9.2 gm per 100 ml, white blood cells 4,800 per cu mm; NPN was normal.

Course in hospital: Temperature continued to be 102° to 104°. Patient became extremely depressed, disoriented, and had hallucinations and refused to eat. She finally became stuporous, temperature rose to 105°, and hemoglobin dropped to 4.2 gm. On the thirtieth day after admission she died. Postmortem examination showed 300 ml of pleural fluid bilaterally, acute esophagitis, small areas of lymphocytic infiltration in the myocardium, and some congestion of capillary tufts of the glomeruli.

The first two attacks in this patient responded well to a conservative regimen. In the third and fatal attack she had severe infection in addition to "lupus crisis." Steroid treatment played no role in this infection.

Case 10 (Fig. A 10). This 16-year-old white man was first admitted in November 1955 with a complaint of fever and severe pain on breathing of 1 week's duration. One year before he had developed a bright red rash on his cheeks which lasted for 1 month. Four months before admission he had two episodes of fever, chills, and headache lasting 10 days. Soon thereafter the rash recurred on his face, he noted fatiguability and had stiffness and swelling of knees, elbows, and fingers. Two months before admission, chills, fever and increased joint symptoms were treated with "2 pills" of cortisone daily. Two weeks later he developed chills, fever of 102°, and pleuritic pain and was given tetracycline. One week before admission he developed cough with rusty sputum. He was admitted to another hospital where he was "treated for pneumonia" with penicillin and tetracycline hydrochloride (Achromycin) with decrease in temperature from 104° to normal, and was given 10 mg of prednisone 4 times a day. On admission to the M.G.H. examination showed an acutely ill man with bilateral chest pain, dyspnea and orthopnea; temperature 105°, pulse 150, BP 100/70, respirations 34; a maculopapular rash in butterfly distribution; heart negative; dullness, and decreased breath sounds and tactile fremitus over the lower half of the chest on both sides; liver dullness 1 cm below the costal margin; spleen palpable 2 cm below the costal margin. Laboratory examination showed 4 + albuminuria, urine loaded with red and white cells and a few granular casts; hemoglobin 11.2 gm/100 ml; leukocyte count 6,050 with 88% neutrophils; chest x-ray showed some pneumonitis. NPN was 54 mg per 100 ml and creatinine 1.24 mg with a clearance of 146 liters in 24 hours. Electrocardiogram showed a PR interval of 0.22 with a rate of 94. Sputum culture showed abundant Staphylococcus aureus. Sedimentation rate was 1.32 mm per min. On a regime of strict bed rest, chloramphenicol (chloromycetin) 500 mg, q.6 h., erythromycin 500 mg, q.6 h., aspirin 0.6 gm 5 i.d. and cortisone 100 mg, q.6 h., he improved rapidly and was free of symptoms

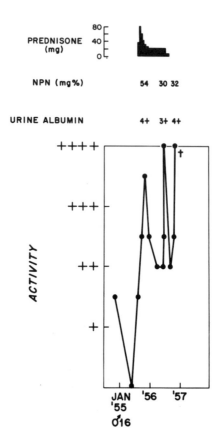

Figure A10. Course of systemic lupus erythematosus from onset in case 10. The symbols +, + +, + + +, and + + + + indicate arbitrary estimates of the total activity of the disease. This patient received steroids as indicated.

in 2 weeks. The cortisone dose was lowered slowly but steadily and he was discharged after 8 weeks in the hospital, free of symptoms except for some fatigue and on a dose of 120 mg of cortisone daily. Three months later, pleuritic chest pain, fever of 100°, and cough productive of a small amount of yellow sputum developed. He was readmitted to the hospital. Physical examination remained approximately the same except for Cushingoid characteristics. Sputum culture again showed Staphylococcus aureus. Urine showed 3+ albumin, 50-60 red cells, and 25-30 white cells per high-power field. Hemoglobin was 8.5 gm per 100 ml. NPN was 30 mg per 100 ml. Psychosis with refusal to take medicine and some paranoid ideas developed. Nephrotic syndrome with serum albumin of 1.6 gm per 100 ml was apparent. Temperature rose to 103°. On a regimen of chloramphenicol, erythromycin, aspirin, and cortisone 50 mg q.12 h. he improved slowly. After 6 weeks the recurrent episodes of

fever of 104° and symptoms subsided, with the exception of numerous paresthesias in legs. Four weeks later he was discharged on aspirin 9.0 gm and cortisone 25 mg a day.

Four weeks after discharge weakness and pains in chest recurred and gradually increased, and 4 weeks later he was readmitted to the hospital. Physical
examination showed temperature 102°. There was increased wasting of muscles but little other change.

Urine examination showed 4+ albumin, many granular casts and 20-30
white cells. Hemoglobin was 10 gm per 100 ml. NPN was 32 mg per 100 ml.
Chest x-ray showed development of pleural effusions. Sputum culture showed
abundant Staphylococcus aureus. He became more dyspneic and dehydrated,
coughed up blood, and his condition deteriorated rapidly. Superficial femoral
veins were ligated. On the following day he died—3 weeks after admission
and 2 years after onset of the disease. Postmortem examination demonstrated
extensive bilateral pneumonia, with abscess, and an old healed pulmonary
infarct. There was evidence of diffuse severe SLE and focal necrotizing glomerulitis with "wire-loop" formation.

In this patient, the combination of very severe SLE and a persistent staphy-
lococcal pulmonary infection were uncontrollable.

Cases 11 and 12 manifested courses which started with severe disease but subsided to a stage of slight activity or full remission for
many years. Case 11 was treated with aspirin as the only anti-inflammatory drug; case 12 received cortisone during the periods of severe
activity of the disease.

Case 11 (Fig. A 11). This 43-year-old white woman was first admitted on July
4, 1947, with a complaint of skin rash, vomiting, chills and fever of 5 days'
duration. For 10-15 years she had developed skin lesions following exposure
to sunlight. Eleven days before admission, she had several long exposures to
sun and 6 days later she developed skin rash and recurrent vomiting. On
examination she was acutely ill. Temperature was 104°, pulse 100, BP 100/70.
There was erythema and hyperpigmentation of skin of face and arms; residues
of vesicles on arms and back; petechial lesions on forearms and mucous membranes of mouth, cervical and axillary lymphadenopathy. Laboratory findings were: urine normal except for + to + + albumin; hemoglobin 9.4 gm per
100 ml; leukocyte count 3,200 per high-power field with 80% neutrophils;
NPN was 56 mg per 100 ml; chest x-ray showed a few small areas of increased
density. On a regimen of penicillin and transfusions every day or two, she
remained acutely ill, disoriented, or semicomatose; incontinent of feces and
urine; temperature rose to 106° and she became icteric. The course was complicated by the development of bilateral gluteal abscesses that were drained.
After 6 weeks she began to improve and condition improved steadily to discharge on November 19. She improved slowly during the following year, but
the right gluteal abscess continued to drain. She was readmitted in December

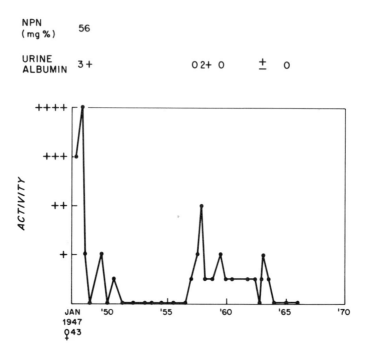

Figure A11. Course of systemic lupus erythematosus from onset in case 11. The symbols +, + +, + + + and + + + + indicate arbitrary estimates of the total activity of the disease. This patient was treated conservatively.

1948 for excision of the sinus. Following discharge, she continued to do very well for the next 8½ years. Then she developed fatigue, a rash on one finger, increasing weakness, and urinary frequency. She was readmitted in November 1957. Examination showed an erythematous papular rash on arms, legs, and feet. Laboratory findings were: urine with 2+ albumin and positive culture for E. coli; hemoglobin 11.4 gm per 100 ml; leukocyte count 3,250 per cu mm with 51% neutrophils. NPN was 28 mg per 100 ml. Creatinine clearance was 91 liters in 24 hours. On a regimen of bed rest, tetracycline hydrochloride, methenamine mandelate, and hydroxychloroquine, she improved steadily, and was discharged in 3 weeks. She continued to do well.

After the series ended, she developed Hodgkin's lymphoma in 1970 and died in 1972.

This patient with very severe SLE responded slowly on a conservative regimen, and the disease went into complete remission for 8½ years. There was no apparent renal involvement.

Case 12 (Fig. A 12). This 15-year-old white girl was admitted in September 1950 with a complaint of loss of appetite. Four months previously, she had noted weakness, anorexia, ulcerations in her mouth, and she had a fever of

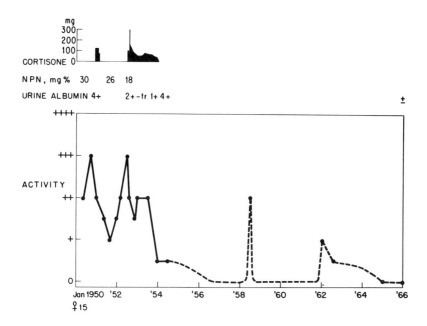

Figure A12. Course of systemic lupus erythematosus from onset in case 12. The symbols +, + +, + + +, and + + + + indicate arbitrary estimates of the total activity of the disease. This patient was treated with steroids as indicated.

104°. These symptoms persisted and she lost 50 pounds. Examination showed temperature 102° rectally, pulse 100, and BP 118/85. She was cachectic, listless, and apprehensive. Skin was coarse, thickened, and scaling; lips were cracked; trunk and ankles were pigmented. Laboratory examination showed: urine with 4 + albumin, 1-2 granular casts and 1 red-cell cast; hemoglobin 5.0 gm per 100 ml; leukocyte count 5,500 with 76% neutrophils; sedimentation rate 1.1 mm per min; no LE cells; NPN 30 mg per 100 ml; and serum albumin 3.0 gm per 100 ml and globulin 4.7 gm. Chest x-ray showed a small left pleural effusion and moderate cardiac enlargement. Electrocardiogram showed flat T waves.

Course: The diagnosis remained unknown. On a regimen of bed rest and occasional transfusions, her condition remained the same except for increasing depression. After 2 months, cortisone was started in a dose of 25 mg, 5 times a day. Slow improvement occurred but small joint effusions appeared in left elbow and knees. After 3 months in the hospital, she was discharged on 75 mg of cortisone a day. However, 6 days later, on December 26, 1950, she was readmitted because of increased dullness in left axilla. Examination remained unchanged except for palpable liver, 3 cm below the costal margin. Urine contained 2 + albumin and rare granular casts; hemoglobin was 10.3 gm per 100 ml; leukocyte count 6,700. NPN was 24 mg per 100 ml. Cortisone was discontinued slowly over 10 days, and she was given 6 transfusions. She improved gradually, gained 6 pounds, and was discharged after 3 weeks. Following discharge, she continued to feel well and gained 20 pounds, but slight cardiac enlargement and pleural effusion persisted for 6 months. Albuminuria of 2+ persisted. Hemoglobin was 8.5 gm. Eleven months after discharge, a rash with much crusting appeared on face and ears, and she had nonproductive cough. She was admitted for the third time in January 1952. Examination showed temperature 99°, pulse 88, BP 116/84; a crusted, weeping rash around eyes and ears, and scaly, erythematous lesions on forehead, arms, and trunk. Laboratory findings were: urine with + albumin; hemoglobin 10.2 gm per 100 ml; leukocyte count 8,900 per cu mm with 64% neutrophils. NPN was 23 mg per 100 ml. Chest x-ray showed increased density in right lower lobe. LE cells were found. She improved on a regimen of chloramphenicol and bacitracin ointment, and was discharged in 10 days. However, the lesions around face, axillae, and perineum became worse in 1 month and she was readmitted in March 1952. General physical examination was unchanged. Urine albumin was +; hemoglobin 9.7 gm and leukocytes 8,800 per cu mm. The skin lesions continued to spread markedly and showed evidence of superimposed infection. There was improvement in the skin with more intensive local therapy, but general condition deteriorated steadily. After 3 months, cortisone in a dose of 25 mg t.i.d. was started. She continued to have episodes of fever, on one occasion to 104°. With increase of cortisone to 150 mg, her general condition improved. Five months after admission she was discharged on 80 mg of cortisone. She improved steadily and was free of symptoms and rash in 2 months. However, 3 months later she had a head cold, developed a nonproductive cough, and rash recurred around ears. She was readmitted in January 1953. Examination showed scaly rash around ears and over upper chest. On a regimen of 50 mg of ACTH a day added to the cortisone of 50 mg a day, she improved and was discharged in 10 days. During the following 3 months, her rash subsided and she felt well for the following year. She was then followed for 12 years by another doctor. During that period she was well except for elevation of blood pressure during one pregnancy, and a period of "anemia" in 1964. When seen here in 1966, she was feeling well and examination was negative. Urine showed ± albumin; hemoglobin was 10.8 gm per 100 ml; leukocyte count 6,200 per cu mm; sedimentation rate 0.41 mm per min.

She has continued to feel well.

After approximately four years of moderately active SLE, the disease went into remission, which persisted for 12 years. She was treated with repeated hospitalizations and steroids.

Cases 13 and 14 illustrate courses of mild activity for years, followed by severe exacerbations resulting in death. Case 13 was treated with aspirin only, case 14 received prednisone in moderate doses for the last 4 months.

Case 13 (Fig. A 13). This 17-year-old white woman was first admitted to the hospital in 1940 with a complaint of cold, blue, moist hands. She had always had cool, moist hands and feet but 1 year before admission noted that her hands were purple with dark red blotches after exposure to cold. Her hands and feet remained cold and purple all of the time. Past history was negative. Physical examination showed temperature of 98° orally, pulse 80, BP 126/88. Hands and feet were cold, moist, and had spotty areas of cyanosis. Laboratory examination showed urine normal; leukocyte count 5,400 per cu mm with 70% neutrophils; hemoglobin 70%; chest x-ray was negative.

Course: Left and right dorsal sympathectomies were performed 2 weeks apart. Following each operation temperature rose to 102° for two days. Hands became warm and pink immediately after operation but symptoms in feet became worse. Six and one-half years later she developed a rash over nose, cheeks, arms, and legs. She was treated with penicillin, sulfathiazole, and bismuth injections. Within 2 hours a rash developed over entire face, and she had a stomatitis and conjunctivitis. Fever continued for 3 months. Hands again became cold and blue. She was given a second course of sulfonamides, followed in 4 days by an exacerbation of the rash on chest, back, and arms. Subsequently, she had malaise, fatigue, and anorexia and was admitted to another hospital in September 1947. Physical examination showed temperature 99°; pulse 80; BP 116/85; circular, erythematous, scaling lesions on face, neck, chest, back, and palms. Urine examination was normal; electrocardiogram was within normal limits; chest x-ray was normal. Hemoglobin was 9.9 gm per 100 ml; leukocyte count was 5,950 with 67% neutrophils; platelets were 375,000 per cu mm; sedimentation rate was 60 mm/hr.

Following discharge she continued to have the rash and fatigue. When seen in the outpatient clinic 3 months later, the rash was unchanged and hands and feet were cold and cyanotic. On a regimen of rest and aspirin she improved and returned to work 4 months later. She felt quite well but hands and feet

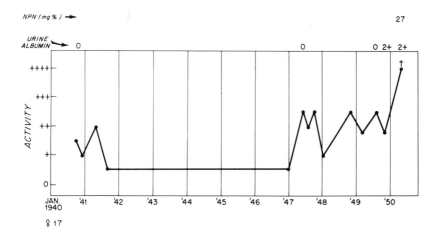

Figure A13. Course of systemic lupus erythematosus from onset in case 13. The symbols +, + +, + + +, and + + + + indicate arbitrary estimates of the total activity of the disease. This patient was treated conservatively.

were cold and blue. Four months later she developed joint pain and swelling of knees, ankles, feet, hands, and elbows, and noted marked fatigue. Occasionally rash recurred on her face. Examination was negative except for cold, moist, cyanotic hands and feet, and slight swelling of the proximal phalangeal joints. Hemoglobin was 11.8 gm per 100 ml, leukocyte count 7,800; sedimentation rate 1.38 mm per min; and urine was negative. She stopped work and felt better for 1 month but then developed retrosternal and left chest pain. This improved with increased bed rest. She again felt fairly well for 4 months, but then noted increased fatigue, recurrence of the rash, and slight fever. She was admitted to another hospital and her course was steadily downhill to death in 4 months. Postmortem examination showed wire-loop changes in the glomeruli, "onion skin" fibrosis around splenic vessels; extensive focal hepatic necrosis; and pleural and pericardial adhesions.

This patient had mild disease for 7 years. Thereafter the disease became more severe and she died 3 years later. The increased activity started after two courses of sulfonamide therapy, to each of which she had a reaction.

Case 14 (Fig. A 14). This 16-year-old white woman was first admitted in October 1949 with a complaint of pain in upper abdomen. Six months before admission she had fever, joint pains, and easy fatiguability; after 2 months she was admitted to another hospital and treated with bed rest and penicillin; she improved gradually though she continued to lose weight. She remained free of symptoms until 5 days before admission to the M.G.H., when she developed sudden onset of pain in the left upper quadrant, radiating to the chest. Examination showed temperature 100.8°, pulse 100, BP 95/60; spleen tender and enlarged, reaching to the umbilicus; lymphadenopathy in posterior cervical region; pain and slight limitation of motion in metacarpophalangeal joints, wrists, elbows, and shoulders. Laboratory findings were: hemoglobin 9.0 gm per 100 ml; leukocyte count 950 per cu mm, falling later to 450; neutrophils 36%. Urine showed 1 to 2+ albumin and occasional red cells; serum albumin was 3.4 gm per 100 ml and globulin 3.1 gm; NPN was 24 mg per 100 ml. Synovial fluid showed good mucin precipitate, and a leukocyte count of 600. Erythrocyte sedimentation rate was 1.8 mm per min. Electrocardiogram was normal except for inverted T_1 and T_2 waves. LE cells were not seen. Serum hemolytic complement was 74 (normal 80-140). Chest and abdominal x-rays were negative except for the enlarged spleen. On a regimen of bed rest, aspirin 0.6 gm/q.3 h. and repeated transfusions, she improved slowly and was discharged after 4 months. She continued to improve with less fatiguability and fewer joint pains, and remained fairly well for almost 7 years. During this period she received small doses of steroids. Spleen was removed in 1953. She was admitted to another hospital in November 1956 because of slight swelling of her face. She was treated with 40 mg of prednisone daily.

In March 1957 she was admitted to the M.G.H. for the second time. For 1 month she had had a cough productive of yellow sputum, and gradually had increasing difficulty in breathing. When seen by her physician 6 days before admission the prednisone was stopped entirely. Examination on admission showed a severely ill patient with moderate respiratory distress, temperature 100.6° rectally, pulse 84, respiration 40; BP 98/85. Heart was enlarged;

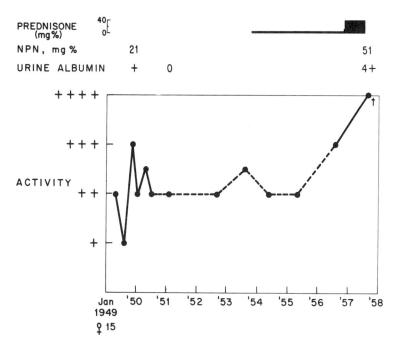

Figure A14. Course of systemic lupus erythematosus from onset in case 14. The symbols +, ++, +++, and ++++ indicate arbitrary estimates of the total activity of the disease. This patient was treated with steroids as indicated.

sounds were good but an inconstant gallop was present. Lungs showed dullness and rales at both bases. Eyelids were very puffy with purple discoloration. There was generalized lymphadenopathy. Joints showed deforming arthritis of hands with ulnar deviation and flexion deformities of elbows. There was moderate ankle edema. Laboratory findings: urine showed 4+ albumin, and was loaded with granular casts; hemoglobin 13.7 gm per 100 ml; leukocyte count 9,850 per cu mm; NPN was 51 mg per 100 ml; sputum culture showed Staphylococcus aureus; chest x-ray showed bilateral pleural effusions; electrocardiogram showed low voltage and inverted $T_{2,3}$, AVFV $_{2-6}$; serum albumin was 1.7 gm per 100 ml; globulin 3.4 gm; NPN 71 mg per 100 ml. She was treated with prednisone 30 mg a day, increased to 100 mg, and chloramphenicol and erythromycin and salt-free albumin, but her condition became much worse. Pericardial tap yielded only 25 ml. She developed severe chest pain and became oliguric, and died on the eighth day. Postmortem examination showed focal pulmonary hemorrhage and bronchopneumonia; hemopericardium; thrombosis of right auricle; chronic passive congestion of the liver; and healed pleuritis.

In the first severe attack the patient improved slowly on a conservative regimen and remained quite well for 7 years. The final attack was apparently precipitated by a respiratory infection. The severity of the attack was increased by the sudden omission of prednisone.

Cases 15 and 16 demonstrate a type of course that starts with mild disease, then has a severe exacerbation, followed by mild disease for years. Case 15 received only aspirin, case 16 was treated with moderate or small doses of steroids.

Case 15 (Fig. A 15). This 68-year-old white woman was first admitted in July 1961 because of skin rash on face and arms, fever and "footdrop." She had been in good health except for asthma and various drug allergies, and arthritis in both knees for 4 years. Four and one-half months before admission, 9 days after an injection of tetanus antitoxin, she developed chills, fever of 101°, fatigue, and pain and swelling of her legs from the knees down. Six weeks before admission a rash appeared on her face, shoulders, and arms, and 4 weeks later she noted "foot drop" and numbness of hands and feet. She lost 15 pounds. Examination showed temperature 99°, pulse 100, and BP 120/80. There were patches of erythema, telangectasia and plugging on face, neck, and arms. On the lower legs was symmetrical petechial eruption. The parotid glands were slightly enlarged. Laboratory examination showed urine normal except for

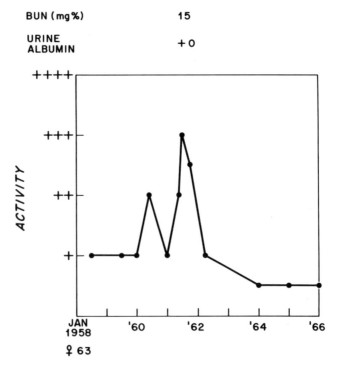

Figure A15. Course of systemic lupus erythematosus from onset in case 15. The symbols +, + +, + + +, and + + + + indicate arbitrary estimates of the total activity of the disease. This patient was treated conservatively.

occasional + albuminuria; hemoglobin 9.9 gm per 100 ml; leukocyte count 4,050 per cu mm; reticulocyte count 3.9%; Coomb's test negative; BUN 15 mg per 100 ml; serum albumin 3.7 gm and globulin 3.8 gm per 100 ml; γ globulin increased; LE test negative; latex fixation test for rheumatoid arthritis positive; electrocardiogram normal. Skin biopsy was consistent with lupus; there was some perivascular infiltration. Neurological examination was normal. It was thought by some observers that the weakness of dorsiflexion of the ankles was due to the painful arthritis rather than to neurological abnormality. On a regimen of bed rest and aspirin she improved steadily and was discharged in 3 weeks. During the following 6 months she became free of all symptoms except for slight dryness of her mouth. She was leading a normal life without medication.

She has continued to do well since the series ended.

This patient had mild disease at the onset, with a subsequent exacerbation perhaps precipitated by injection of tetanus antitoxin. The attack subsided quickly and the disease went into remission.

Case 16 (Fig. A 16). This 50-year-old white woman was first admitted in 1959. Two and one-half years previously she had facial rash and arthralgias. Laboratory examination at that time had shown urine negative, a low leukocyte count, elevated sedimentation rate, and positive LE cell test. She was treated with prednisone, 10 to 20 mg a day, with good response. Prednisone dosage was reduced slowly. In 4 months she was free of symptoms and labo-

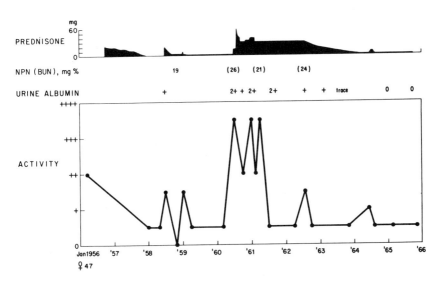

Figure A16. Course of systemic lupus erythematosus from onset in case 16. The symbols +, ++, +++, and ++++ indicate arbitrary estimates of the total activity of the disease. This patient was treated with steroids as indicated.

ratory tests were normal. She remained free of symptoms for 5 months after prednisone was discontinued. Because of recurrence of arthralgias and rash, she was treated with triamcinolone. The dosage of 16 mg was steadily reduced to 2 to 4 mg and she remained free of symptoms for the 5 months preceding admission. One hour before admission severe anterior chest pain developed. Physical examination showed temperature 101°, pulse 76, BP 118/78. She was in acute distress, and restless, but examination otherwise was negative. Laboratory findings were: hemoglobin 12.7 gm per 100 ml; leukocyte count 8,300 per cu mm with 64% neutrophils; urine showed + albumin; NPN was 19 mg per 100 ml. Electrocardiogram showed changes of acute, anterior septal myocardial infarction; chest x-ray was negative, no LE cells were seen. She improved steadily and was discharged in 10 weeks.

Dosage of triamcinolone (Aristocort) had been increased to 8 mg a day following the myocardial infarction but had been reduced to 4 mg at the time of discharge. She remained free of all symptoms for 2½ months, when arthralgias recurred. Two weeks later, anterior chest pain "different than the coronary pain" developed, and she had chills and fever of 102°. Examination showed a pericardial rub. Laboratory findings were unchanged. Chest x-ray showed some atelectasis of left lower lobe. Electrocardiogram showed changes in the T waves in the mid-precordial leads consistent with pericarditis. She improved rapidly and was discharged in 5 days. During the following week, she had nausea, vomiting, and malaise, and noted some arthralgias. Triamcinolone had been continued at a dose of 8 to 12 mg per day. Because of recurrent nausea, vomiting, and malaise she was readmitted for the third time in July 1960. Examination showed temperature 101° rectally, pulse 110, BP 120/80; laboratory findings were urine with 2+ albumin, 18-20 leukocytes, and granular casts; hemoglobin 11.8 gm per 100 ml; leukocyte count 9,000 per cu mm with 81% neutrophils; BUN 26 mg per 100 ml; creatinine 1.1 mg per 100 ml with a clearance of 46 liters in 24 hours; many LE cells; sedimentation rate of 52 mm per hr; electrocardiogram showed only the pattern of old anterior myocardial infarction; chest x-ray showed some pleural thickening on the left. On the day following admission a pleural rub was heard on the right and subsequently a pleural effusion developed. She remained acutely ill for 4 weeks and then improved slowly and was discharged after 2 months on 32 mg of prednisone. However, 3 months later she was readmitted because of severe abdominal pain. On examination she appeared acutely ill. The abdomen was exquisitely tender in the right lower quadrant. At operation a perforation of the terminal ileum was found. Following closure of the perforation she improved rapidly. Laboratory findings on this admission showed a urinary tract infection with coliform bacilli that responded quickly to treatment. BUN was 21 mg per 100 ml, hemoglobin 13.8 gm per 100 ml, leukocyte count 15,300 with 81% neutrophils. After 2 weeks she was discharged, free of symptoms. She continued a dose of 40 mg of prednisone with gradual reduction to 24 mg. She continued to be free of symptoms for 18 months, when she developed headache, malaise, cough, and discomfort in the chest. She was readmitted and examination showed Cushingoid features, and rales at bases. X-ray of chest showed acute patchy infiltration of left lower lobe. Urine showed + + albumin; BUN was 24 mg per 100 ml; hematocrit was 37% leukocyte count was 14,000 with 64% neutrophils. Electrocardiogram showed only evidence of an old anteroseptal infarct. She improved rapidly on penicillin treatment and was discharged in 1 week. She continued to take 24 mg of methylprednisolone. Subsequently, she remained free of symptoms and worked regularly. After the series was closed she continued to do well for 6 years, when she had a perforation of a diverticulum of the colon. Again she recovered very well, but 8 months later had perforation of the right colon and died.

In this patient there were two severe exacerbations, one associated with myocardial infarction, and the other with perforation of the terminal ileum. On a regimen of hospitalizations and steroid therapy she recovered and the disease went into good remission for over 10 years.

Case 17 represents a course in which there was no evidence of renal involvement during the first attack, but fatal renal failure in a second attack 22 months later.

Case 17 (Fig. A 17). This 16-year-old white girl was admitted in July 1944 with a complaint of chest pain of 5 days' duration. Two years before admission, she began to have pain and swelling in one or another finger, recurring every few weeks. Six months later she began to have recurrent pain in the left knee, and subsequently in the feet. Three months before admission, she had an upper respiratory infection with laryngitis and for 3 days pain in left axilla. The chest pain recurred 5 days before admission and she developed fever. Examination showed: temperature 101°; pulse 100; BP 95/65; enlarged anterior cervical and right supraclavicular nodes; and a small area of dullness in left axilla. Laboratory findings showed: urine normal except for + albumin on one occasion; hemoglobin 12 gm per 100 ml; leukocyte count 7,400 per cu mm with 66% neutrophils; sedimentation rate 0.82 mm per min; NPN 29 mg per 100 ml. Chest x-ray showed some increased density in the anterior portion of the left lower lobe and some pleural fluid. No evidence of tuberculosis was obtained. On a regimen of bed rest and aspirin, she became free of symptoms and was sent to a tuberculosis hospital after 2 months for continued bed rest. The diagnosis was thought by most to be SLE or RA. She became entirely free of symptoms, felt well, and returned to school 2 months after discharge from the sanitorium. She continued to do well for 18 months, when she noted dark brown urine, swelling of her ankles, some exertional dyspnea, headache, and vomiting. On admission to another hospital, examination showed temperature 100°, pulse 100, respiration 22, and BP 130/70. Heart was slightly enlarged, and there was slight edema of ankles. Laboratory findings were: urine brown with 4+ albumin, loaded with red cells and a few white cells and casts; hemoglobin 11.6 gm per 100 ml; leukocyte count 4,400 with 65% neutrophils; sedimentation rate 0.98 mm per min; BUN 40 mg per 100 ml; serum albumin 1.8 gm and globulin 2.5 gm per 100 ml, and electrocardiogram was normal. Soon after admission she developed a butterfly rash. The course was intermit-

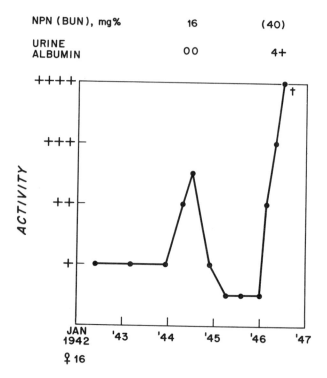

Figure A17. Course of systemic lupus erythematosus from onset in case 17. The symbols +, ++, +++, and ++++ indicate arbitrary estimates of the total activity of the disease. This patient was treated conservatively.

tently downhill; BUN rose to 120 mg per 100 ml and she died 7 weeks after admission.

In this case there was no suggestion during the first attack of the severe renal involvement that developed after 22 months.

Bibliography   Index

Bibliography

The bibliography contains only references pertinent to this book. A more complete bibliography is given by Dubois [70].

1. Ackerman, G.L. Alternate-day steroid therapy in lupus nephritis, *Ann. Intern. Med.* 72:511-519, 1970.
2. Adams, D.A., Gordon, A., and Maxwell, M.H. Azathioprine treatment of immunological renal disease, *J.A.M.A.* 199:459-463, 1967.
3. Alarcón-Segovia, D. Drug-induced lupus syndromes, *Mayo Clin. Proc.* 44:664-681, 1969.
4. Alarcón-Segovia, D., Galbraith, R.F., Maldonado, J.E., and Howard, F.M. Jr. Systemic lupus erythematosus following thymectomy for myasthenia gravis, *Lancet* 2:662-665, 1963.
5. Alarcón-Segovia, D., Herskòvic, T., Dearing, W.H., Bartholomew, L.G., Cain, J.C., and Shorter, R.G. Lupus erythematosus cell phenomenon in patients with ulcerative colitis, *Gut* 6:39-47, 1965.
6. Alarcón-Segovia, D., Khalil, G.W., Worthington, J.W., and Ward, L.E. Clinical and experimental studies on the hydralazine syndrome and its relationship to systemic lupus erythematosus, *Medicine* 46:1-33, 1967.
7. Alarcón-Segovia, D., and Osmundson, P.J. Peripheral vascular syndromes associated with systemic lupus erythematosus, *Ann. Intern. Med.* 62:907-919, 1965.
8. Andreasen, J.O. Oral manifestations in discoid and systemic lupus erythematosus: I. Clinical investigation, *Acta Odontol. Scand.* 22:295-310, 1964.
9. Ansell, B.M., and Lawrence, J.S. A family study in lupus erythematosus (abstract), *Arthritis Rheum.* 6:260, 1963.
10. Arana, R., and Seligmann, M. Antibodies to native and denatured deoxyribonucleic acid in systemic lupus erythematosus, *J. Clin. Invest.* 46:1867-1882, 1967.
11. Armas-Cruz, R., Harnecker, J., Ducach, G. Jalil, J., and Gonzalez, F. Clinical diagnosis of systemic lupus erythematosus, *Am. J. Med.* 25:409-419, 1958.
12. Arnett, F.C., Bias, W.B., and Shulman, L. Studies in familial systemic lupus erythematosus (abstract), *Arthritis Rheum.* 15:102-103, 1972.
13. Asboe-Hansen, G. A survey of the normal and pathological occurrence of mucinous substances and mast cells in the dermal connective tissue in man, *Acta Derm. Venereol.* 30:338-347, 1950.
14. Atkins, C.J., Kondon, J.J. Jr., Quismorio, F.P., and Friou, G.J. The choroid plexus in systemic lupus erythematosus, *Ann. Intern. Med.* 76:65-72, 1972.
15. Baehr, G., Klemperer, P., and Schifrin, A. A diffuse disease of the peripheral circulation usually associated with lupus erythematosus and endocarditis, *Trans. Assoc. Am. Physicians* 50:139-155, 1935.
16. Baggenstoss, A.H. Visceral lesions in disseminated lupus erythematosus, *Proc. Staff Meet. Mayo Clin.* 27:412-419, 1952.
17. Bain, G.O. The pathology of Mikulicz-Sjögren disease in relation to disseminated lupus erythematosus: A review of the autopsy findings and presentation of a case, *Can. Med. Assoc. J.* 82:143-148, 1960.

18. Baldwin, D.S., Lowenstein, J., Rothfield, N.F., Gallo, G., and Mc-Cluskey, R.T. The clinical course of the proliferative and membranous forms of lupus nephritis, *Ann. Intern. Med.* 73:929-942, 1970.

19. Barnett, E.V. Diagnostic aspects of lupus erythematosus cells and antinuclear factors in disease states, *Mayo Clin. Proc.* 44:645-648, 1969.

20. Barnett, E.V., North, A.F. Jr., Condemi, J.J., Jacox, R.F., and Vaughan, J.H. Antinuclear factors in systemic lupus erythematosus and rheumatoid arthritis, *Ann. Intern. Med.* 63:100-108, 1965.

21. Baš, H., and Vachtenheim, J. Neurologische Erscheinungen beim systematischen Lupus erythematodes, *Dtsch. Z. Nervenheilkunde* 185:244-251, 1963.

22. Bauer, F.K., Riley, W.C., and Cohen, E.B. Disseminated lupus erythematosus with Syndenham's chorea and rheumatic heart disease: Report of a case with autopsy, *Ann. Intern. Med.* 33:1042-1053, 1950.

23. Baum, J., and Ziff, M. Decreased 19S antibody response to bacterial antigens in systemic lupus erythematosus, *J. Clin. Invest.* 48:758-767, 1969.

24. Bennett, J.C., Claybrook, J., Kinsey, H., and Holley, H.L. The clinical manifestations of systemic lupus erythematosus, *J. Chronic Dis.* 13:411-425, 1961.

25. Bennett, J.C., Osment, L.S., and Holley, H.L. Immunologic manifestations of a group of patients with a diagnosis of discoid lupus erythematosus, *Arthritis Rheum.* 4:490-497, 1961.

26. Benton, J.W., Tynes, B., Register, H.B. Jr., Alford, C., and Holley, H.L. Systemic lupus erythematosus occurring during anticonvulsive drug therapy, *J.A.M.A.* 180:115-118, 1962.

27. Berg, P., Postel, A.H., and Lee, S.L. Perforation of the ileum in steroid-treated systemic lupus erythematosus: a case report, *Am. J. Dig. Dis.* 5:274-282, 1960.

28. Berlyne, G.M., Short, I.A., and Vickers, C.F.H. Placental transmission of the L.E. factor, *Lancet* 2:15-17, 1957.

29. Bernhard, G.C., Lange, R.L., and Hensley, G.T. Aortic disease with valvular insufficiency as the principal manifestation of systemic lupus erythematosus, *Ann. Intern. Med.* 71:81-87, 1969.

30. Bloch, K.J., and Bunim, J.J. Sjögren's syndrome and its relation to connective tissue diseases, *J. Chronic Dis.* 16:915-927, 1963.

31. Bloch, K.J., and Helms, C.M. Antinuclear antibodies. The value of immunofluorescence patterns and titers, *Mass. Gen. Hosp. Newsletter* 6, No. 2, 1973.

32. Bishko, F. Retinopathy in systemic lupus erythematosus. A case report and review of the literature, *Arthritis Rheum.* 15:57-63, 1972.

33. Blomgren, S.E., Condemi, J.J., Bignall, M.C., and Vaughan, J.H. Antinuclear antibody induced by procainamide, *N. Engl. J. Med.* 281:64-66, 1969.

34. Bollet, A.J. The intrinsic viscosity of synovial fluid hyaluronic acid, *J. Lab. Clin. Med.* 48:721-728, 1956.

35. Bowie, E.J.W., Thompson, J.H. Jr., Pascuzzi, C.A., and Owen, C.A. Jr. Thrombosis in systemic lupus erythematosus despite circulating anticoagulants, *J. Lab. Clin. Med.* 62:416-430, 1963.

36. Brandt, K.D., Cathcart, E.S., and Cohen, A.S. Studies of immune deposits in synovial membranes and corresponding synovial fluids, *J. Lab. Clin. Med.* 72:631-647, 1968.

37. Bridge, R.G., and Foley, F.E. Placental transmission of the lupus erythematosus factor, *Am. J. Med. Sci.* 227:1-8, 1954.

38. Brigden, W., Bywaters, E.G.L., Lessof, M.H., and Ross, I.P. The heart in systemic lupus erythematosus, *Br. Heart J.* 22:1-16, 1960.

39. Brown, C.H., Scanlon, P.J., and Haserick, J.R. Mesenteric arteritis with perforation of the jejunum in a patient with systemic lupus erythematosus, *Cleve. Clin. Q.* 31:169-178, 1964.

40. Brunjes, S., Zike, K., and Julian, R. Familial systemic lupus erythematosus: A review of the literature with a report of ten additional cases in four families, *Am. J. Med.* 30:529-536, 1961.

41. Burnham, T.K., Neblett, T.R., and Fine, G. The application of the fluorescent antibody technic to the investigation of lupus erythematosus and various dermatoses, *J. Invest. Dermatol.* 41:451-456, 1963.

42. Cammarata, R.J., Rodnan, G.P., and Crittenden, J.O. Systemic lupus erythematosus with chorea, *J.A.M.A.* 184:971-973, 1963.

43. Carr, R.E., Henkind, P., Rothfield, N., and Siegel, I.M. Ocular toxicity of antimalarial drugs, *Am. J. Ophthalmol.* 66:738-744, 1968.

44. Casals, S.P., Friou, G.J., and Teague, P.O. Specific nuclear reaction pattern of antibody to DNA in lupus erythematosus sera, *J. Lab. Clin. Med.* 62:625-631, 1963.

45. Cass, R.M., Mongan, E.S., Jacox, R.F., and Vaughan, J.H. Immunoglobulins G, A, and M in systemic lupus erythematosus: Relationship to serum C' titer, latex titer, ANA and manifestations of clinical disease, *Ann. Intern. Med.* 69:749-756, 1968.

46. Castro, O., Farber, L.R., and Clyne, L.P. Circulating anticoagulants against Factors IX and XI in systemic lupus erythematosus, *Ann. Intern. Med.* 77:543-548, 1972.

47. Cheatum, D.E., Hurd, E.R., Strunk, S.W., and Ziff, M. Renal histology and clinical course of systemic lupus erythematosus, *Arthritis Rheum.* 16:670-676, 1973.

48. Clark, E.C., and Bailey, A.A. Neurological and psychiatric signs associated with systemic lupus erythematosus, *J.A.M.A.* 160:455-457, 1956.

49. Coburn, A.F., and Moore, D.H. The plasma proteins in disseminated lupus erythematosus, *Johns Hopkins Hosp. Bull.* 73:196-221, 1943.

50. Cohen, A.S., and Calkins, E. A controlled study of chloroquine as an antirheumatic agent, *Arthritis Rheum.* 1:297-312, 1958.

51. Cohen, A.S., Reynolds, W.E., Franklin, E.C., Kulka, J.P., Ropes, M.W., Shulman, L.E., and Wallace, S.L. Preliminary criteria for the classification of systemic lupus erythematosus, *Bull. Rheum. Dis.* 21:643-648, 1971.

52. Cohen, P., and Gardner, F.H. Sulfonamide reactions in systemic lupus erythematosus, *J.A.M.A.* 163:817-819, 1966.

53. Comerford, F.R., and Cohen, A.S. The nephropathy of systemic lupus erythematosus, *Medicine* 46:425-473, 1967.

54. Conference on effects of chronic salicylate administration. U.S. Dept. of Health, Education, and Welfare, Bethesda, Maryland, 1966.

55. Cook, C.D., Wedgwood, R.J.P., Craig, J.M., Hartmann, J.R., and Janeway, C.A. Systemic lupus erythematosus (description of 37 cases in children and a discussion of endocrine therapy in 32 of the cases), *Pediatrics* 26:570-585, 1960.

56. Cooperating Clinics Committee of the American Rheumatism Association. A seven-day variability study of 499 patients with peripheral rheumatoid arthritis, *Arthritis Rheum.* 8:302-335, 1965.

57. Copeland, G.D., von Capeller, D., and Stern, T.N. Systemic lupus erythematosus: A clinical report of 47 cases with pathologic findings in 18, *Am. J. Med. Sci.* 236:318-325, 1958.

58. Cormane, R.H. "Bound" globulin in the skin of patients with chronic discoid lupus erythematosus and systemic lupus erythematosus, *Lancet* 1:534-535, 1964.

59. Crosnier, J., Slama, R., and deMontera, H. Les Lupoérythémato-néphrites: I. Etude clinique et anatomique de quatorze observations, *Presse Med.* 68:148-151, 1960.

60. Cross, R.J. Systemic lupus erythematosus: combined staff clinics of College of Physicians and Surgeons, Columbia Univ. and Presbyt. Hospital, *Am. J. Med.* 28:416-429, 1960.

61. Cruickshank, B. Lesions of joint and tendon sheaths in systemic lupus erythematosus, *Ann. Rheum. Dis.* 18:111-119, 1959.

62. Daly, D. Central nervous system in acute disseminate lupus erythematosus, *J. Nerv. Ment. Dis.* 102:461-465, 1945.

63. Dameshek, W., and Reeves, W.H. Exacerbation of lupus erythematosus following splenectomy in "idiopathic" thrombocytopenic purpura and autoimmune hemolytic anemia, *Am. J. Med.* 21:560-566, 1956.

64. Dameshek, W., and Schwartz, R. Treatment of certain "autoimmune" diseases with antimetabolites; a preliminary report, *Trans. Assoc. Am. Physicians* 73:113-127, 1960.

65. Domz, C.A., McNamara, D.H., and Holzapfel, H.F. Tetracycline provocation in lupus erythematosus, *Ann. Intern. Med.* 50:1217-1226, 1959.

66. Donadio, J.V. Jr., Holley, K.E., Wagoner, R.D., Ferguson, R.H., and McDuffie, F.C. Treatment of lupus nephritis with prednisone and combined prednisone and azathioprine, *Ann. Intern. Med.* 77:829-835, 1972.

67. Dubois, E.L. The effect of the L.E. cell test on the clinical picture of systemic lupus erythematosus, *Ann. Intern. Med.* 38:1265-1294, 1953.

68. Dubois, E.L. Nitrogen mustard in treatment of systemic lupus erythematosus, *Arch. Intern. Med.* 93:667-672, 1954.

69. Dubois, E.L. Lupus Erythematosus: A Review of the Current Status of Discoid and Systemic Lupus Erythematosus and Their Variants, McGraw-Hill Book Company, New York, 1966.

70. Dubois, E.L. Lupus Erythematosus: A Review of the Current Status of Discoid and Systemic Lupus Erythematosus, 2d ed. University of Southern California Press, Los Angeles, Calif. 1974.

71. Dubois, E.L. Procainamide induction of a systemic lupus erythematosus-like syndrome, *Medicine* 48:217-228, 1969.

72. Dubois, E.L., Horowitz, R.E., Demopoulos, H.B., and Teplitz, R.

NZB/NZW mice as a model of systemic lupus erythematosus, *J.A.M.A.* 195: 285-289, 1966.

73. Dustan, H.P., Taylor, R.D., Corcoran, A.C., and Page, I.H. Rheumatic and febrile syndrome during prolonged hydralazine treatment, *J.A.M.A.* 154:23-29, 1954.

74. Duthie, J.J.R. Discussion, in Levy, G., Biopharmaceutical aspects of the gastrointestinal absorption of salicylates, *in* A. St. J. Dixon, B.K. Martin, M.J.H. Smith, and P.H.N. Wood (eds.), Salicylates, an International Symposium, p. 17, J. and A. Churchill, Ltd., London, 1963.

75. Eisenberg, H., Dubois, E.L., Sherwin, R.P., and Balchum, O.J. Diffuse interstitial lung disease in systemic lupus erythematosus, *Ann. Intern. Med.* 79:37-45, 1973.

76. Elliott, J.A. Jr., and Mathieson, D.R. Complement in disseminated (systemic) lupus erythematosus, *Arch. Dermatol. Syphilol.* 68:119-128, 1953.

77. Epstein, H.C., and Litt, J.Z. Discoid lupus erythematosus in a newborn infant, *N. Engl. J. Med.* 265:1106-1107, 1961.

78. Estes, D., and Christian, C.L. The natural history of systemic lupus erythematosus by prospective analysis, *Medicine* 50:85-95, 1971.

79. Friedberg, C.K., Gross, L., and Wallach, K. Nonbacterial thrombotic endocarditis associated with prolonged fever, arthritis, inflammation of serous membranes and widespread vascular lesions, *Arch. Intern. Med.* 58:662-684, 1936.

80. Friedman, E.A., and Rutherford, J.W. Pregnancy and lupus erythematosus, *Obstet. Gynecol.* 8:601-609, 1956.

81. Friedman, I.A., Sickley, J.F., Poske, R.M., Black, A., Bronsky, D., Hartz, W.H. Jr., Feldhake, C., Reeder, P.S., and Katz, E.M. The L.E. phenomenon in rheumatoid arthritis, *Ann. Intern. Med.* 46:1113-1136, 1957.

82. Gallo, R.C., and Forde, D.L. Familial chronic discoid lupus erythematosus and hypergammaglobulinemia, *Arch. Intern. Med.* 117:627-631, 1966.

83. Garcia-Morteo, O., Franklin, E.C., McEwen, C., Phythyon, J., and Tanner, M. Studies of relatives of patients with systemic lupus erythematosus, *Arthritis Rheum.* 4:356-363, 1961.

84. Garsenstein, M., Pollak, V.E., and Kark, R.M. Systemic lupus erythematosus and pregnancy, *N. Engl. J. Med.* 267:165-169, 1962.

85. Gary, N.E., Maher, J.F., and Schreiner, G.E. Lupus nephritis: Renal function after prolonged survival, *N. Engl. J. Med.* 276:73-78, 1967.

86. Glaser, G.H. Lesions of the central nervous system in disseminated lupus erythematosus, *A.M.A. Arch. Neurol. Psychiat.* 67:745-753, 1952.

87. Gonzalez, E.N., and Rothfield, N.F. Immunoglobulin class and pattern of nuclear fluorescence in systemic lupus erythematosus, *N. Engl. J. Med.* 274:1334-1338, 1966.

88. Good, R.A. Discussion in Holman, H.R., Genetic studies of SLE, *Arthritis Rheum.* 6:513-523, 1963.

89. Goodman, H.C. Current studies on the effect of antimetabolites in nephrosis, other non-neoplastic diseases, and experimental animals, *Ann. Intern. Med.* 59:388-407, 1963.

90. Griffith, G.C., and Vural, I.L. Acute and subacute disseminated lupus

erythematosus: A correlation of clinical and postmortem findings in eighteen cases. *Circulation* 3:492-500, 1951.

91. Grimley, P.M., Decker, J.L., Michelitch, H.J., and Frantz, M.M. Abnormal structures in circulating lymphocytes from patients with systemic lupus erythematosus and related diseases. *Arthritis Rheum.* 16:313-323, 1973.

92. Gross, L. The heart in atypical verrucous endocarditis (Libman-Sacks), *in* Contributions to the Medical Sciences in Honor of Dr. Emanuel Libman, by His Pupils, Friends and Colleagues, vol. 2, pp. 527-550, International Press, New York, 1932.

93. Gross, L. The cardiac lesions in Libman-Sacks disease (with a consideration of its relationship to acute diffuse lupus erythematosus), *Am. J. Pathol.* 16:375-408, 1940.

94. Grupper, C. Lupus érythémateux familial, 12 cas dans 6 familles, *Sem. Hôp.* 18/4, 1104-1110, 1965.

95. Gueft, B., and Laufer, A. Further cytochemical studies in systemic lupus erythematosus, *Arch. Pathol.* 57:201-226, 1954.

96. Györkey, F., Min, K.W., Sincovics, J.G., and Györkey, P. Systemic lupus erythematosus and myxovirus, *N. Engl. J. Med.* 280:333, 1969.

97. Hadida, M.E., Coulier, L., and Savag, J. Lupus érythémateux chronique avec néphrite: Les Confins du LEC et du LEA, *Bull. Soc. Fr. Dermatol. Syphiligr.* 70:912, 1963.

98. Hadler, N.M., Gerwin, R.D., Frank, M.M., Whitaker, J.N., Baker, M., and Decker, J.L. The fourth component of complement in the cerebrospinal fluid in systemic lupus erythematosus, *Arthritis Rheum.* 16:507-521, 1973.

99. Hahn, B.H., Yardley, J.H., and Stevens, M.B. "Rheumatoid" nodules in systemic lupus erythematosus, *Ann. Intern. Med.* 72:49-58, 1970.

100. Hall, A.P., Bardawil, W.A., Bayles, T.B., Mednis, A.D., and Galins, N. The relations between the antinuclear, rheumatoid and L.E.-cell factors in the systemic rheumatic diseases, *N. Engl. J. Med.* 263:769-775, 1960.

101. Hargraves, M.M., Richmond, H., and Morton, R. Presentation of two bone marrow elements: the "tart" cell and the "L.E." cell, *Proc. Staff Meet. Mayo Clin.* 23:25-28, 1948.

102. Harvey, A.M., Shulman, L.E., Tumulty, P.A., Conley, C.L., and Schoenrich, E.H. Systemic lupus erythematosus: Review of the literature and clinical analysis of 138 cases, *Medicine* 33:291-437, 1954.

103. Haserick, J.R. Modern concepts of systemic lupus erythematosus: Review of 126 cases, *J. Chronic Dis.* 1:317-334, 1955.

104. Haserick, J.R. Six years' survival in severe systemic lupus erythematosus, *Arch. Dermatol.* 75:706-714, 1957.

105. Haserick, J.R., and Corcoran, A.C. ACTH and cortisone in the acute crisis of systemic lupus erythematosus, *J.A.M.A.* 146:643-645, 1951.

106. Hejtmancik, M.R., Wright, J.C., Quint, R., and Jennings, F.L. The cardiovascular manifestations of systemic lupus erythematosus, *Am. Heart J.* 68:119-130, 1964.

107. Heptinstall, R.H., and Sowry, G.S.C. Peripheral neuritis in systemic lupus erythematosus, *Br. Med. J.* 1:525-527, 1952.

108. Hijmans, W., Doniach, D., Roitt, I.M., and Holborrow, E.J. Serological overlap between lupus erythematosus and rheumatoid arthritis, and thyroid autoimmune disease, *Br. Med. J.* 2:909-914, 1961.

109. Hill, L.C. Systemic lupus erythematosus, *Br. Med. J.* 2:655-660 and 726-732, 1957.

110. Hollander, J.L., Jessar, R.A., and McCarty, D.J. Synovianalysis: An aid in arthritis diagnosis, *Bull. Rheum. Dis.* 12:263-264, 1961.

111. Honey, S. Systemic lupus erythematosus presenting with sulphonamide hypersensitivity reaction, *Br. Med. J.* 1:1272-1275, 1956.

112. Hughes, G.R.V., Cohen, S.A., and Christian, C.L. Anti-DNA activity in systemic lupus erythematosus, *Ann. Rheum. Dis.* 30:259-264, 1971.

113. Hughes, G.R.V., Cohen, S.A., Lightfoot, R.W. Jr., Meltzer, J.I., and Christian, C.L. The release of DNA into serum and synovial fluid, *Arthritis Rheum.* 14:259-266, 1971.

114. Humphreys, E.M. The cardiac lesions of acute disseminated lupus erythematosus, *Ann. Intern. Med.* 28:12-14, 1948.

115. Hunicker, L.G., Ruddy, S., Carpenter, C.B., Schur, P.H., Merrill, J.P., Muller-Eberhard, H.J., and Austen, K.F. Metabolism of third complement component (C3) in nephritis, *N. Engl. J. Med.* 287:835-840, 1972.

116. Jackson, R. Discoid lupus in a newborn infant of a mother with lupus erythematosus, *Pediatrics* 33:425-430, 1964.

117. Jacobs, J.C. Systemic lupus erythematosus in childhood. (Report of 35 cases, with discussion of 7 apparently induced by anticonvulsant medication, and of prognosis and treatment.) *Pediatrics* 32:257-264, 1963.

118. James, T.N., Rupe, C.E., and Monto, R.W. Pathology of the cardiac conduction system in systemic lupus erythematosus, *Ann. Intern. Med.* 63:402-410, 1965.

119. Jessar, R.A., Lamont-Havers, R.W., and Ragan, C. Natural history of lupus erythematosus disseminatus, *Ann. Intern. Med.* 38:717-731, 1953.

120. Johnson, H.M. Effect of splenectomy in acute systemic lupus erythematosus, *Arch. Dermatol. Syphilol.* 68:699-713, 1953.

121. Johnson, R.T., and Richardson, E.P. The neurological manifestations of systemic lupus erythematosus, *Medicine* 47:337-369, 1968.

122. Joseph, R.R., and Zarafoneitis, C.J.D. Fatal systemic lupus erythematosus in identical twins: Case reports and review of the literature, *Am. J. Med. Sci.* 249:190-199, 1965.

123. Kacaki, J.N., Callerame, M.L., Blomgren, S.E., and Vaughan, J.H. Immunoglobulin G subclasses of antinuclear antibodies and renal deposits: Comparison of systemic lupus erythematosus, drug induced lupus and rheumatoid arthritis, *Arthritis Rheum.* 14:276-282, 1971.

124. Kalliomaki, J.L., and Hakonen, P. Antibody levels to parainfluenza, herpes simplex, varicella-zoster, cytomegalic virus, and measles virus in patients with connective tissue diseases, *Ann. Rheum. Dis.* 31:192-195, 1972.

125. Kaplan, S.R., and Calabresi, P. Drug therapy: Immunosuppressive agents, *N. Engl. J. Med.* 289:1234-1236, 1973.

126. Kaposi, M.K. Neue Beiträge zur Kenntniss des Lupus erythematosus. *Arch. Dermatol. Syphilol.* 4:36-78, 1872.

127. Keil, H. Conception of lupus erythematosus and its morphologic variants (with particular reference to "systemic" lupus erythematosus), *Arch. Dermatol. Syphilol.* 36:729-757, 1937.

128. Kellum, R.E., and Haserick, J.R. Systemic lupus erythematosus: A statistical evaluation of mortality based on a consecutive series of 299 patients, *Arch. Intern. Med.* 113:200-207, 1964.

129. Kierland, R.R. Classification and cutaneous manifestations of lupus erythematosus, *Proc. Staff Meet. Mayo Clin.* 15:675-677, 1940.

130. Kim, H.H., and Williams, T.J. Endometrioid carcinoma of the uterus and ovaries associated with immunosuppressive therapy and anticoagulation, *Mayo Clin. Proc.* 47:39-41, 1972.

131. Klemperer, P., Pollack, A.D., and Baehr, G. Pathology of disseminated lupus erythematosus, *Arch. Pathol.* 32:569-631, 1941.

132. Klemperer, P., Pollack, A.D., and Baehr, G. Diffuse collagen disease. Acute disseminated lupus erythematosus and diffuse scleroderma, *J.A.M.A.* 119:331-332, 1942.

133. Klinge, F. Der Rheumatismus, *Ergeb. Allg. Pathol. Pathol. Anat.* 27:1-351, 1933.

134. Koffler, D., Schur, P.H., and Kunkel, H.G. Immunological studies concerning the nephritis of systemic lupus erythematosus, *J. Exp. Med.* 126:607-624, 1967.

135. Kong, T.Q., Kellum, R.E., and Haserick, J.R. Clinical diagnosis of cardiac involvement in systemic lupus erythematosus, *Circulation* 26:7-11, 1962.

136. Kraak, J.H., van Ketel, W.G., Prakken, J.R., and van Zwet, W.R. The value of hydroxychloroquine (plaquenil) for the treatment of chronic discoid lupus erythematosus: double blind trial. *Dermatologica* 130:293-305, 1965.

137. Kraus, S.J., Haserick, J.R., and Lantz, M.A. Fluorescent treponemal antibody absorption test reactions in lupus erythematosus, *N. Engl. J. Med.* 282:1287-1290, 1970.

138. Kraus, S.J., Haserick, J.R., and Lantz, M.A. Atypical FTA-ABS test fluorescence in lupus erythematosus patients, *J.A.M.A.* 211:2140-2141, 1970.

139. Kunkel, H.G. Case records of the Massachusetts General Hospital, Case no. 18-1969, *N. Engl. J. Med.* 280:1009-1017, 1969.

140. Kurlander, D.J., and Kirsner, J.B. The association of chronic "nonspecific" inflammatory bowel disease with lupus erythematosus, *Ann. Intern. Med.* 60:799-813, 1964.

141. Kurnick, N.B. A rational therapy of systemic lupus erythematosus, *Arch. Intern. Med.* 97:562-575, 1956.

142. Kushniruk, W. Systemic involvement in chronic lupus erythematosus, *Can. Med. Assoc. J.* 76:184-193, 1957.

143. LaBelle, A., and Tornaben, J.A. Effects of various analgesics on inflammatory edema resulting from silver nitrate injection, *Science* 114:187-189, 1951.

144. Labowitz, R., and Schumacher, H.R. Jr. Articular manifestations of systemic lupus erythematosus, *Ann. Intern. Med.* 74:911-921, 1971.

145. Lange, K., Ores, R., Strauss, W., and Wachstein, M. Steroid therapy of systemic lupus erythematosus based on immunologic considerations, *Arthritis Rheum.* 8:244-259, 1965.

146. Larson, D.L. Systemic Lupus Erythematosus, Little, Brown and Co., Boston, 1961.

147. Lebowitz, W.B. The heart in rheumatoid arthritis (rheumatoid disease): A clinical and pathological study of sixty-two cases, *Ann. Intern. Med.* 58:102-123, 1963.

148. Lenoch, F., and Vojtíšek, O. The prevalence of LE cells in 1,000 consecutive patients with active rheumatoid arthritis, *Acta Rheumatol. Scand.* 13:313-319, 1967.

149. Leonhardt, T. Family studies in systemic lupus erythematosus, *Acta Med. Scand. Suppl.* 416:1-156, 1964.

150. Levy, J., Barnett, E.V., MacDonald, N.S., and Klinenberg, J.R. Altered immunoglobulin metabolism in systemic lupus erythematosus and rheumatoid arthritis, *J. Clin. Invest.* 49:708-715, 1970.

151. Lewis, B.I., Sinton, D.W., and Knott, J.R. Central nervous system involvement in disorders of collagen, *Arch. Intern. Med.* 93:315-327, 1954.

152. Lewis, D.C. Systemic lupus and polyneuropathy, *Arch. Intern. Med.* 116:518-522, 1965.

153. Libman, E., and Sacks, B. A hitherto undescribed form of valvular and mural endocarditis, *Arch. Intern. Med.* 33:701-737, 1924.

154. Lie, T.H., and Rothfield, N.F. An evaluation of the preliminary criteria for the diagnosis of systemic lupus erythematosus, *Arthritis Rheum.* 15:532-534, 1972.

155. Lightfoot, R.W. Jr., and Lotke, P.A. Osteonecrosis of metacarpal heads in systemic lupus erythematosus, *Arthritis Rheum.* 15:486-492, 1972.

156. Lincoln, M., and Ricker, W.A. A case of periarteritis nodosa with L.E. cells; apparent complete remission with cortisone therapy, *Ann. Intern. Med.* 41:639-646, 1954.

157. Lipsmeyer, E.A. Development of malignant cerebral lymphoma in a patient with systemic lupus erythematosus treated with immunosuppression, *Arthritis Rheum.* 15:183-186, 1972.

158. Lowman, E.W., and Slocumb, C.H. The peripheral vascular lesions of lupus erythematosus, *Ann. Intern. Med.* 36:1206-1216, 1952.

159. Mackay, I.R. The clinical features, pathogenesis and therapy of systemic lupus erythematosus, *Med. J. Aust.* 2:279-282, 1958.

160. Mackay, I.R., Eriksen, N., Motulsky, A.G., and Volwiler, W. Cryo- and macroglobulinemia: Electrophoretic, ultracentrifugal, and clinical studies, *Am. J. Med.* 20:564-587, 1956.

161. Mackay, I.R., Goldstein, G., and McConchie, I.H. Thymectomy in systemic lupus erythematosus, *Br. Med. J.* 2:792-793, 1963.

162. Madsen, J.R., and Anderson, G.V. Lupus erythematosus and pregnancy, *Obstet. Gynecol.* 18:492-494, 1961.

163. Maher, J.F., and Schreiner, G.E. Treatment of lupus nephritis with azathioprine, *Arch. Intern. Med.* 125:293-298, 1970.

164. Mäkelä, T.E., Ruosteenoja, R., Wager, O., Wallgren, G.R., and Jokinen, E.J. Myasthenia gravis and systemic lupus erythematosus, *Acta Med. Scand.* 175:777-780, 1964.

165. Malamud, N., and Saver, G. Neuropathologic findings in disseminated lupus erythematosus, *Arch. Neurol. Psychiat.* 71:723-731, 1954.

166. Mandema, E., Pollak, V.E., Kark, R.M., and Rezaian, J. Quantitative observations on antinuclear factors in systemic lupus erythematosus, *J. Lab. Clin. Med.* 58:337-352, 1961.

167. Margolius, A. Jr., Jackson, D.P., and Ratnoff, O.D. Circulating anticoagulants: A study of 40 cases and a review of the literature, *Medicine* 40: 145-202, 1961.

168. Martin, J.R., Wilson, C.L., and Mathews, W.H. Bilateral rupture of ligamenta patellae in a case of disseminated lupus erythematosus, *Arthritis Rheum.* 6:548-552, 1958.

169. Maumenee, A.E. Retinal lesions in lupus erythematosus, *Am. J. Ophthalmol.* 23:971-981, 1940.

170. McAdam, L., Paulus, H.E., and Peter, J.B. Adenocarcinoma of the lung during azathioprine therapy, *Arthritis Rheum.* 17:92-94, 1974.

171. McCuistion, C.H., and Schoch, E.P. Jr. Possible discoid lupus erythematosus in newborn infant, *Arch. Dermatol. Syphilol.* 70:782-785, 1954.

172. McDevitt, D.G., and Glasgow, J.F.T. Lupus-like syndrome induced by procainamide: A case report, *Br. Med. J.* 3:780-781, 1967.

173. Medical Research Council. Treatment of systemic lupus erythematosus with steroids, *Br. Med. J.* 2:915-920, 1961.

174. Mellors, R.C., and Huang, C.Y. Immunopathology of NZB/BL mice V.: Virus-like (filtrable) agent separable from lymphoma cells and identifiable by electron microscopy, *J. Exp. Med.* 124:1031-1038, 1966.

175. Mellors, R.C., Ortega, L.G., and Holman, H.R. Role of gamma globulins in pathogenesis of renal lesions in systemic lupus erythematosus and chronic membranous glomerulonephritis with an observation on the lupus erythematosus cell reaction, *J. Exp. Med.* 106:191-202, 1957.

176. Merrell, J., and Shulman, L.E. Determination of prognosis in chronic disease, illustrated by systemic lupus erythematosus, *J. Chronic Dis.* 1:12-32, 1955.

177. Meyer zum Büschenfeld, K.H., and Springmann, L. Beitrag zur Ätiologie und Pathogenese des erythematodes acutus anhand einer Beobachtung bei einem 4 Monate alte Säugling, *Arch. Klin. Exp. Dermatol.* 216:101-114, 1963.

178. Michael, A.F., Vernier, R.L., Drummond, K.N., Levitt, J.I., Herdman, R.C., Fish, A.J., and Good, R.A. Immunosuppressive therapy of chronic renal disease, *N. Engl. J. Med.* 276:817-828, 1967.

179. Michael, S.R., Vural, I.L., Bassen, F.A., and Schaefer, L. The hematologic aspects of disseminated (systemic) lupus erythematosus, *Blood* 6:1059-1072, 1951.

180. Milne, J.A., Anderson, J.R., MacSween, R.N., Fraser, K., Short, I.,

Stevens, J., Shaw, G.B., and Tankel, H.I. Thymectomy in acute systemic lupus erythematosus and rheumatoid arthritis, *Br. Med. J.* 1:461-464, 1967.

181. Miyasato, F., Pollak, V.E., and Barcelo, R. Serum B_1A (B_1C) globulin levels in systemic lupus erythematosus: Their relationship to clinical and renal histologic findings, *Arthritis Rheum.* 9:308-317, 1966.

182. Moffitt, G.R. Jr. Complete atrioventricular dissociation with Stokes-Adams attacks due to disseminated lupus erythematosus, *Ann. Intern. Med.* 63:508-511, 1965.

183. Montgomery, H., and McCreight, W.G. Disseminate lupus erythematosus, *Arch. Dermatol. Syphilol.* 60:356-372, 1949.

184. Mook, W.H., Weiss, R.S., and Bromberg, L.K. Lupus erythematosus disseminatus, *Arch. Dermatol. Syphilol.* 24:786-829, 1931.

185. Moore, J.E., and Lutz, W.B. The natural history of systemic lupus erythematosus: An approach to its study through chronic biologic false positive reaction, *J. Chron. Dis.* 1:297-316, 1955.

186. Mortensen, V., and Gormsen, H. Lupus erythematosus disseminatus (Libman-Sacks' disease), *Acta Med. Scand. Suppl.* 266:743-774, 1952.

187. Muehrcke, R.C., Kark, R.M., Pirani, C.L., and Pollak, V.E. Lupus nephritis: a clinical and pathologic study based on renal biopsies, *Medicine* 36:1-145, 1957.

188. Mund, A., Simson, J., and Rothfield, N. Effect of pregnancy on course of systemic lupus erythematosus, *J.A.M.A.* 183:917-920, 1963.

189. Myers, E.N., Bernstein, J.M., and Fostiropolous, G. Salicylate ototoxicity: A clinical study, *N. Engl. J. Med.* 273:587-590, 1965.

190. Myers, E.N., and Bernstein, J.M. Salicylate ototoxicity: A clinical and experimental study, *Arch. Otolaryngol.* 82:483-493, 1965.

191. Myers, A.N., and Mills, J.A. Personal communication.

192. Nice, C.M. Jr. Congenital disseminated lupus erythematosus, *Am. J. Roentgenol.* 88:585-587, 1962.

193. Noonan, C.D., Odone, D.T., Engleman, E.P., and Splitter, S.D. Roentgenographic manifestations of joint disease in systemic lupus erythematosus, *Radiology* 80:837-843, 1963.

194. O'Connor, J.F., and Musher, D.M. Central nervous system involvement in systemic lupus erythematosus, *Arch. Neurol.* 14:157-164, 1966.

195. Osler, W. On the visceral manifestations of the erythema group of skin diseases, *Am. J. Med. Sci.* 127:1-23, 1904.

196. Paradise, J.L. Sydenham's chorea without evidence of rheumatic fever: Report of its association with the Henoch-Schönlein syndrome and with systemic lupus erythematosus, and review of the literature, *N. Engl. J. Med.* 263:625-629, 1960.

197. Paull, A.M. Occurrence of the "L.E." phenomenon in a patient with a severe penicillin reaction, *N. Engl. J. Med.* 252: 128-129, 1955.

198. Pekin, T.J. Jr., and Zvaifler, N.J. Synovial fluid findings in systemic lupus erythematosus (SLE), *Arthritis Rheum.* 13:777-785, 1970.

199. Petz, L.D., Sharp, G.C., Cooper, N.R., and Irvin, W.S. Serum and cerebral spinal fluid complement and serum autoantibodies in systemic lupus erythematosus, *Medicine* 50:259-275, 1971.

200. Phillips, J.C., and Howland, W.J. Mesenteric arteritis in systemic lupus erythematosus, *J.A.M.A.* 206:1569-1570, 1968.

201. Pincus, T., Schur, P.H., Rose, J.A., Decker, J.L., and Talal, N. Measurement of serum DNA-binding activity in systemic lupus erythematosus, *N. Engl. J. Med.* 281:701-705, 1969.

202. Pohle, E.L., and Tuffanelli, D.L. Study of cutaneous lupus erythematosus by immunohistochemical methods, *Arch. Dermatol.* 97:520-526, 1968.

203. Pollak, V.E., Grove, W.J., Kark, R.M., Muehrcke, R.C., Pirani, C.L., and Steck, I.E. Systemic lupus erythematosus simulating acute surgical condition of the abdomen, *N. Engl. J. Med.* 259:258-266, 1958.

204. Pollak, V.E., Pirani, C.L., and Schwartz, F.D. The natural history of the renal manifestations of systemic lupus erythematosus, *J. Lab. Clin. Med.* 63:537-550, 1964.

205. Purnell, D.C., Baggenstoss, A.H., and Olsen, A.M. Pulmonary lesions in disseminated lupus erythematosus, *Ann. Intern. Med.* 42:619-628, 1955.

206. Reiches, A.J. The lupus erythematosus syndrome: The relationship of discoid (cutaneous) lupus erythematosus to systemic (disseminated) lupus erythematosus, *Ann. Intern. Med.* 46:678-684, 1957.

207. Rodnan, G.P., Maclachlan, M.J., and Creighton, A.S. Study of serum proteins and serologic reactions in relatives of patients with S.L.E. (abstract), *Clin. Res.* 8:197, 1960.

208. Ropes, M.W. Observations on the natural course of disseminated lupus erythematosus, *Medicine* 43:387-391, 1964.

209. Ropes, M.W. The relationship of salicylate levels to toxicity at various ages (abstract), *Excerpta Med. Found. Int. Cong. Ser. N.*, 167, 1967.

210. Ropes, M.W., and Bauer, W. Synovial Fluid Changes in Joint Disease, Harvard University Press, Cambridge, Mass., 1953.

211. Rose, G.A. An unusual clinical recovery from systemic lupus erythematosus, *Ann. Rheum. Dis.* 20:289-292, 1961.

212. Rothfield, N.F. Alertness to symptoms of impending flare-up held systemic lupus erythematosus management key, *Clin. Trends Rheumatol.* 4:1-4, 1970.

213. Rothfield, N., March, C.H., Miescher, P., and McEwen, C. Chronic discoid lupus erythematosus, *N. Engl. J. Med.* 269:1155-1161, 1963.

214. Rothfield, N.F., McCluskey, R.T., and Baldwin, D.S. Renal disease in systemic lupus erythematosus, *N. Engl. J. Med.* 269:537-544, 1963.

215. Rothfield, N.F., and Pace, N. Relation of positive L.E.-cell preparations to activity of lupus erythematosus and corticosteroid therapy, *N. Engl. J. Med.* 266:535-538, 1962.

216. Rothfield, N.F., Phythyon, J.M., McEwen, C., and Miescher, P. The role of antinuclear reactions in the diagnosis of SLE: A study of 53 cases, *Arthritis Rheum.* 4:223-239, 1961.

217. Rourke, M.D., and Ernstene, A.C. A method for correcting the erythrocyte sedimentation rate for variations in the cell volume percentage of blood, *J. Clin. Invest.* 8:545-559, 1930.

218. Rowe, P.B. Disseminated lupus erythematosus with Sydenham's

chorea: Report of a case with a review of the literature, *Med. J. Aust.* 2:586-588, 1963.

219. Ruderman, M., and McCarty, D.J. Aseptic necrosis in systemic lupus erythematosus: Report of a case involving six joints, *Arthritis Rheum.* 7:709-721, 1964.

220. Rupe, C.E., and Nickel, S.N. New clinical concept of systemic lupus erythematosus, *J.A.M.A.* 171:1055-1061, 1959.

221. Russell, P.W., Haserick, J.R., and Zucker, E.M. Epilepsy in systemic lupus erythematosus, *Arch. Intern. Med.* 88:78-92, 1951.

222. Scarpelli, D.G., McCoy, F.W., and Scott, J.K. Acute lupus erythematosus with laryngeal involvement, *N. Engl. J. Med.* 261: 691-694, 1959.

223. Scheinberg, L. Polyneuritis in systemic lupus erythematosus, *N. Engl. J. Med.* 255:416-421, 1956.

224. Schoenfeld, M.R., and Messeloff, C.R. Cardiac tamponade in systemic lupus erythematosus, *Circulation* 27:98-99, 1963.

225. Schur, P.H., and Austen, K.F. Complement in the rheumatic diseases, *Bull. Rheum. Dis.* 22:666-673, 1971-1972.

226. Schur, P.H., and Sandson, J. Immunologic factors and clinical activity in systemic lupus erythematosus, *N. Engl. J. Med.* 278:533-538, 1968.

227. Schur, P.H., Stollar, D., Steinberg, A.D., and Talal, N. Incidence of antibodies to double-stranded RNA in systemic lupus erythematosus and related diseases, *Arthritis Rheum.* 14:342-347, 1971.

228. Scott, A., and Rees, E.G. The relationship of systemic lupus erythematosus and discoid lupus erythematosus: A clinical and hematological study, *AMA Arch. Dermatol.* 79:422-435, 1959.

229. Seip, M. Systemic lupus erythematosus in pregnancy with haemolytic anaemia, leucopenia and thrombocytopenia in the mother and her newborn infant, *Arch. Dis. Childhood* 35:364-366, 1960.

230. deSèze, S., Kahn, M.F., Aubert, B., and Solnica, J. Survenue d'une névrite optique au d'un lupus érythémateux, disséminé méconnu: Intérêt de l'enquête familiale, *Bull. Soc. Méd. Hôp. Paris,* 115:1017, 1964.

231. Sharon, E., Kaplan, D., and Diamond, H.S. Exacerbation of systemic lupus erythematosus after withdrawal of azathioprine therapy, *N. Engl. J. Med.* 288:122-124, 1973.

232. Shearn, M.A. The heart in systemic lupus erythematosus, *Am. Heart J.* 58:452-466, 1959.

233. Shearn, M.A., and Pirofsky, B. Disseminated lupus erythematosus, *Arch. Intern. Med.* 90:790-807, 1952.

234. Short, C.L., Bauer, W., and Reynolds, W.E. Rheumatoid Arthritis: A definition of the disease and a clinical description based on a numerical study of 293 patients and controls. Harvard University Press, Cambridge, Mass., 1957.

235. Shulman, H.J., and Christian, C.L. Aortic insufficiency in systemic lupus erythematosus, *Arthritis Rheum.* 12:138-146, 1969.

236. Shulman, L.E. Inducing agents and relationship to other diseases. *In* Immunologic Aspects of Rheumatoid Arthritis and Systemic Lupus Erythematosus, *Arthritis Rheum.* 6:558-571, 1963.

237. Shulman, L.E., and Harvey, A.M. The nature of drug-induced systemic lupus erythematosus (abstract), *Arthritis Rheum.* 3:464, 1960.

238. Siegel, M., Lee, S.L., Widelock, D., Gwon, N.V., and Kravitz, H. A comparative family study of rheumatoid arthritis and systemic lupus erythematosus, *N. Engl. J. Med.* 273:893-897, 1965.

239. Siegel, M., Lee, S.L., Widelock, D., Reilly, E.B., Wise, G.J., Zingale, S.B., and Fuerst, H.T. The epidemiology of systemic lupus erythematosus: Preliminary results in New York City, *J. Chronic Dis.* 15:131-140, 1962.

240. Siguier, F., Godeau, P., Levy, R., Binet, J.L., and Rueff, B. Lupus érythémateux et grossesse, *Bull. Soc. Méd. Hôp. Paris* 115:119, 1964.

241. Siemsen, J.K., Brook, J., and Meister, L. Lupus erythematosus and avascular bone necrosis. A clinical study of three cases and review of the literature, *Arthritis Rheum.* 5:492-501, 1962.

242. Smith, J.F. The kidney in lupus erythematosus, *J. Pathol. Bacteriol.* 70:41-51, 1955.

243. Soffer, L.J. The therapy of systemic lupus erythematosus, *J. Mt. Sinai Hosp. New York* 26:297-306, 1959.

244. Soffer, L.J., Southren, A.L., Weiner, H.E., and Wolf, R.L. Renal manifestations of systemic lupus erythematosus: A clinical and pathologic study of 90 cases, *Ann. Intern. Med.* 54:215-228, 1961.

245. Sokoloff, L. The heart in rheumatoid arthritis, *Am. Heart J.* 45:635-643, 1953.

246. Spaeth, G.L. Corneal staining in systemic lupus erythematosus, *N. Engl. J. Med.* 276:1168-1171, 1967.

247. Stafford, C.T., Niedermeier, W., Holley, H.L., and Pigman, W. Studies in the concentration and intrinsic viscosity of hyaluronic acid in synovial fluids of patients with rheumatic diseases, *Ann. Rheum. Dis.* 23:152-157, 1964.

248. Staples, P.J., Gerding, D.N., Decker, J.L., and Gordon, R.S. Jr. Incidence of infection in systemic lupus erythematosus, *Arthritis Rheum.* 17:1-10, 1974.

249. Stastny, P., and Ziff, M. Cold-insoluble complexes and complement levels in systemic lupus erythematosus, *N. Engl. J. Med.* 280:1376-1381, 1969.

250. Steinberg, A.D. Cytotoxic drugs in treatment of nonmalignant diseases, *Ann. Intern. Med.* 76:619-642, 1972.

251. Steinberg, A.D., Kaltreider, H.B., Staples, P.J., Goetzl, E.J., Talal, N., and Decker, J.L. Cyclophosphamide in lupus nephritis: A controlled trial, *Ann. Intern. Med.* 75:165-171, 1971.

252. Steinberg, A.D., and Talal, N. The coexistence of Sjögren's syndrome and systemic lupus erythematosus, *Ann. Intern. Med.* 74:55-61, 1971.

253. Stenstam, T. On the occurrence of keratoconjunctivitis sicca in cases of rheumatoid arthritis, *Acta Med. Scand.* 127:130-148, 1947.

254. Stewart, M. Personal communication.

255. Stickney, J.M., and Keith, N.M. Renal involvement in disseminated lupus erythematosus, *Arch. Intern. Med.* 66:643-660, 1940.

256. Stollar, D. Reactions of systemic lupus erythematosus sera with histone fractions and histone-DNA complexes, *Arthritis Rheum.* 14:485-492, 1971.

257. Stuart, M.J., Murphy, S., Oski, F.A., Evans, A.E., Donaldson, M.H., and Gardner, F.H. Platelet function in recipients of platelets from donors ingesting aspirin, *N. Engl. J. Med.* 287:1105-1109, 1972.

258. Svanborg, A. and Sölvell, L. Incidence of disseminated lupus erythematosus, *J.A.M.A.* 165:1126-1128, 1957.

259. Sztejnbok, M., Stewart, A., Diamond, H., and Kaplan, D. Azathioprine in the treatment of systemic lupus erythematosus: A controlled study, *Arthritis Rheum.* 14:639-645, 1971.

260. Talal, N., and Steinberg, A.D. Inhibition of anti-DNA antibodies in human and mouse lupus by viral and synthetic ribonucleic acid (abstract), *Arthritis Rheum.* 14:187, 1971.

261. Tan, E.M., and Kunkel, H.G. An immunofluorescent study of the skin lesions in systemic lupus erythematosus, *Arthritis Rheum.* 9:37-46, 1966.

262. Tan, E.M., Schur, P.H., Carr, R.I., and Kunkel, H.G. Deoxyribonucleic acid (DNA) and antibodies to DNA in the serum of patients with systemic lupus erythematosus, *J. Clin. Invest.* 45:1732-1740, 1966.

263. Tannenbaum, H., and Schur, P.H. Development of reticulum cell sarcoma during cyclophosphamide therapy, *Arthritis Rheum.* 17:15-18, 1974.

264. Tatelman, M., and Keech, M.K. Esophageal motility in systemic lupus erythematosus, rheumatoid arthritis, and scleroderma, *Radiology* 86:1041-1046, 1966.

265. Taubenhaus, M., Eisenstein, B., and Pick, A. Cardiovascular manifestations of collagen diseases, *Circulation* 12:903-920, 1955.

266. Thivolet, J., Verjus, F., and Kratchko, A. Les facteurs héréditares dans le Lupus érythémateux disséminé, *Ann. Dermatol. Syphilig. Paris* 91:361, 1964.

267. Thurman, D.L., Toone, E.C. Jr., and Vaughan, J.H. Systemic lupus erythematosus, an increasing problem: A clinical survey of 35 cases, *Va. Med. Mon.* 85:71-74, 1958.

268. Toone, E.C. Jr., Irby, R., and Pierce, E.L. The L.E. cell in rheumatoid arthritis, *Am. J. Med. Sci.* 240:599-608, 1960.

269. Trimble, R.B., Townes, A.S., Robinson, H., Kaplan, S.B., Chandler, R.W., Hanissian, A.S., and Masi, A.T. Preliminary criteria for the classification of systemic lupus erythematosus (SLE): Evaluation in early diagnosed SLE and rheumatoid arthritis, *Arthritis Rheum.* 17:184-188, 1974.

270. Tu, W.H., and Shearn, M.A. Systemic lupus erythematosus and latent renal tubular dysfunction, *Ann. Intern. Med.* 67:100-109, 1967.

271. Tuffanelli, D.L., and Dubois, E.L. Cutaneous manifestations of systemic lupus erythematosus, *Arch. Dermatol.* 90:377-386, 1964.

272. Tuffanelli, D.L., Kay, D., and Fukuyama, K. Dermal-epidermal junction in lupus erythematosus, *Arch. Dermatol.* 99:652-662, 1969.

273. Twining, R.H., Marcus, W.Y., and Garvey, J.L. Tendon rupture in systemic lupus erythematosus, *J.A.M.A.* 189:377-378, 1964.

274. Voegele, G.E., and Dietze, H.J. Neuropsychiatric symptoms in systemic lupus erythematosus, *P. Psych. Q.* 3:11-18, 1963.

275. Ward, J.R., Cloud, R.S., and Turner, L.M. Jr., Non-cytotoxicity of "nuclear antibodies" from lupus erythematosus sera in tissue cultures, *Ann. Rheum. Dis.* 23:381-388, 1964.

276. Weiss, S., and Mallory, T.B. Case records of the Massachusetts General Hospital, Case no. 24201, *N. Engl. J. Med.* 218:838-845, 1938.

277. Wilkinson, M. Rheumatoid pericarditis: A report of 4 cases, *Br. Med. J.* 2:1723-1726, 1962.

278. Wilson, R.M., Maher, J.F., and Schreiner, G.E. Lupus nephritis: Clinical and histologic survey, *Arch. Intern. Med.* 111:429-438, 1963.

279. Winslow, W.A., Ploss, L.N., and Loitman, B. Pleuritis in systemic lupus erythematosus: its importance as an early manifestation in diagnosis, *Ann. Intern. Med.* 49:70-88, 1958.

280. Wolf, S.M., and Barrows, H.S. Myasthenia gravis and systemic lupus erythematosus, *Arch. Neurol.* 14:254-258, 1966.

281. Wood, P.H.N., Harvey-Smith, E.A., and Dixon, A. St. J. Salicylates and gastrointestinal bleeding: Acetylsalicylic acid and aspirin derivatives, *Br. Med. J.* 1:669-675, 1962.

282. Young, D., and Schwedel, J.B. The heart in rheumatoid arthritis, *Am. Heart J.* 28:1-23, 1944.

283. Yurchak, P.M., Levine, S.A., and Gorlin, R. Constrictive pericarditis complicating disseminated lupus erythematosus, *Circulation* 31:113-118, 1965.

284. Ziff, M. Viruses and the connective tissue diseases, *Ann. Intern. Med.* 75:951-958, 1971.

285. Zingale, S.B., Minzer, L., Rosenberg, B., and Lee, S.L. Drug-induced lupus-like syndrome, *Arch. Intern. Med.* 112:63-66, 1963.

286. Zingale, S.B., Sánchez Avalos, J.C., Andrada, J.A., Stringa, S.G., and Manni, J.A. Appearance of anticoagulant factors and certain "autoimmune" antibodies following antigenic stimulation with blood group substances in patients with systemic lupus erythematosus, *Arthritis Rheum.* 6:581-598, 1963.

287. Zweiman, B.J., Kornblum, J., Cornog, J., and Hildreth, E.A. The prognosis of lupus nephritis: Role of clinical-pathologic correlations, *Ann. Intern. Med.* 69:441-462, 1968.

Index